100 Questions & Answers About Celiac Disease and Sprue

David L. Burns, MD, CNSP, FACG

Department of Gastroenterolog
Lahey Clinic
Burlington, M

JONES AND BARTLETT PUBLISHERS
Sudbury, Massachusetts
BOSTON   TORONTO   LONDON   SINGAPORE

World Headquarters

Jones and Bartlett Publishers	Jones and Bartlett Publishers	Jones and Bartlett Publishers
40 Tall Pine Drive	Canada	International
Sudbury, MA 01776	6339 Ormindale Way	Barb House, Barb Mews
978-443-5000	Mississauga, Ontario L5V 1J2	London W6 7PA
info@jbpub.com	CANADA	UK
www.jbpub.com		

Jones and Bartlett's books and products are available through most bookstores and online booksellers. To contact Jones and Bartlett Publishers directly, call 800-832-0034, fax 978-443-8000, or visit our Web site, www.jbpub.com.

Substantial discounts on bulk quantities of Jones and Bartlett's publications are available to corporations, professional associations, and other qualified organizations. For details and specific discount information, contact the special sales department at Jones and Bartlett via the above contact information or send an email to specialsales@jbpub.com.

The authors, editor, and publisher have made every effort to provide accurate information. However, they are not responsible for errors, omissions, or for any outcomes related to the use of the contents of this book and take no responsibility for the use of the products and procedures described. Treatments and side effects described in this book may not be applicable to all people; likewise, some people may require a dose or experience a side effect that is not described herein. Drugs and medical devices are discussed that may have limited availability controlled by the Food and Drug Administration (FDA) for use only in a research study or clinical trial. Research, clinical practice, and government regulations often change the accepted standard in this field. When consideration is being given to use of any drug in the clinical setting, the health care provider or reader is responsible for determining FDA status of the drug, reading the package insert, and reviewing prescribing information for the most up-to-date recommendations on dose, precautions, and contraindications, and determining the appropriate usage for the product. This is especially important in the case of drugs that are new or seldom used.

Library of Congress Cataloging-in-Publication Data
Burns, David L.
    100 questions and answers about celiac disease and sprue : a Lahey Clinic guide / David L. Burns.
        p. cm.
    Includes index.
    ISBN-13: 978-0-7637-4502-8 (pbk. : alk. paper)
    ISBN-10: 0-7637-4502-2
    1. Celiac disease—Miscellanea. 2. Celiac disease—Popular works. I. Title. II. Title: One hundred questions and answers about celiac disease.
    RC862.C44B87 2008
    616.3'99—dc22
                            2007021388

Production Credits

Executive Publisher: Christopher Davis	Manufacturing Buyer: Therese Connell
Production Director: Amy Rose	Composition: Appingo
Associate Production Editor: Rachel Rossi	Cover Design: Jon Ayotte
Associate Editor: Kathy Richardson	Printing and Binding: Malloy, Inc.
Associate Marketing Manager: Rebecca Wasley	Cover Printing: Malloy, Inc.

6048

Printed in the United States of America
11 10 09 08 07   10 9 8 7 6 5 4 3 2 1

CONTENTS

Foreword   **v**

Preface   **ix**

Acknowledgments   **xi**

Dedication   **xiii**

Part 1: The Basics   **1**

- What is celiac disease?
- Does celiac disease run in families?
- Does celiac disease affect both genders?

Part 2: Symptoms and Manifestations   **13**

- Are there different kinds of celiac disease?
- Can I have celiac disease without any symptoms?
- What is the association between lactose intolerance and celiac disease?

Part 3: Children and Celiac Disease   **51**

- Do children get celiac disease?
- Which diseases are associated with celiac disease in children?
- What are the complications of celiac disease in children?

Part 4: Evaluation and Diagnosis   **69**

- How is celiac disease diagnosed?
- Do I need to see a specialist?
- What are the blood tests for celiac disease?

Part 5: Treatment for Celiac Disease: The Gluten-Free Diet   **105**

- What is gluten?
- What is a gluten-free diet?
- Should I see a dietitian?

Part 6: Management of Celiac Disease   135

- Do I need to stay on a gluten-free diet for life?
- What's next if the diet is not working?
- Do I need any vaccinations?

Part 7: Dermatitis Herpetiformis   155

- What is dermatitis herpetiformis?
- Are there any other skin diseases associated with celiac disease?
- What is the treatment for dermatitis herpetiformis?

Part 8: Diseases Associated with Celiac Disease   161

- What is the association between selective IgA deficiency and celiac disease?
- What is the association between type 1 diabetes and celiac disease?
- What is the association between autoimmune disease and celiac disease?

Part 9: Complications   171

- What are refractory sprue and collagenous sprue?
- What is ulcerative jejunitis?
- What is the relationship between celiac disease and cancer (including lymphoma)?

Part 10: Patient Resources   181

- Are there support groups for celiac disease?
- Where can I get more information on the gluten-free diet?
- What support or information is available for children with celiac disease?

Part 11: Conclusion   189

- What is the future of celiac disease? Will there be a medication that can treat this disease?

Appendix   193

Glossary   195

Index   207

In this book author Dr. David Burns has carefully defined and expertly addressed the many questions asked by those living with celiac disease and by their relatives, friends and colleagues. In order to fully appreciate the value and timeliness of this work it is important to know something of the dramatic transformations that have occurred in recent years regarding our understanding of how celiac disease impacts the population of the United States.

The generally held perception of celiac disease within the medical community in the US prior to 2000 was that of a rare disorder afflicting children with severe diarrhea and failure to thrive, and where clinical improvement on a gluten free diet led to a diagnosis. These attitudes were so widely held that the National Institutes of Health convened a consensus development conference in 2004 to highlight these and other misconceptions surrounding celiac disease. The consensus statement that resulted contradicted each of the points listed above and pointed to recent studies in the US and worldwide that painted a very different picture of the realities of celiac disease.[1] So, let us briefly consider each of these contentious points in turn.

A study performed by a highly respected group of US investigators and published in the widely read *American Journal of Gastroenterology* in 1994 found that approximately 1 in 5,000 (1 in 1:4587 to be more precise)[2] of the population were diagnosed as having celiac disease translating to a total of approximately 61,000 individuals in the US. In the late 1990's powerful new blood tests (endomysial and tissue transglutaminase antibody assays) allowed for more accurate identification of celiac disease in the community. In one study of over 13,000 US Americans the prevalence of celiac disease

---

1. Celiac Disease: Proceedings of the NIH Consensus Conference on Celiac Disease, June 28–30, 2004, Bethesda, MD. *Gastroenterology* 128 (suppl 1):4; 2005.
2. Talley et al, Am J Gastroenterol, 1994.

in those without any evident risk factors was a startling 0.75%.[3] This was more that thirty-fold greater than the 1994 estimate and predicted a US celiac population of over 2 million. Almost immediately celiac disease was transformed from a rare to a common disorder. Most experts believe that the celiac "epidemic" results from increased awareness and improved detection rather than any dramatic increase in true prevalence of the disease.

The myth that celiac disease primarily presents in early childhood is contradicted by numerous recent studies indicating that the peak age of celiac disease diagnosis in the US is not in 4-year-olds but in those in their 40s.[4] Similarly, the so called classic presentation of severe diarrhea, weight loss and overt malabsorption is unusual. Most patients present with mild gastrointestinal symptoms that are easily mistaken for irritable bowel syndrome or accepted by long term suffers and their physicians as a variant of normal or as just "a sensitive stomach." An even greater source of diagnostic error is when celiac disease presents with disorders outside of the gastrointestinal tract such as thinning of the bones (osteoporosis), reduced fertility, skin rash (dermatitis herpetiformis) or nervous system disorders. In fact, the single most common presentation of celiac disease in the US is with anemia caused by iron malabsorption that often arises in the complete absence of any gastrointestinal complaints whatsoever.

Finally, the common misconception that celiac disease is best diagnosed by monitoring changes in symptoms on a gluten-free diet has led to a myriad of misdiagnoses. Some with celiac disease did not respond promptly, leading to the correct diagnosis being abandoned. More commonly, a non-specific or placebo response to the major dietary changes inherent in switching to a gluten- free diet has led many Americans to needlessly adhere to this challenging lifelong dietary regimen. Everyone who understands the nuances of celiac disease and the gluten-free diet agree that the objective markers of an increase in endomysial or tissue transglutaminase antibody concentrations in the blood and the findings of characteristic intestinal injury in biopsies

3. Fasano A, Berti I, Gerarduzzi T, et al. Prevalence of celiac disease in at-risk and not-at-risk groups in the United States: a large multicenter study. Arch Intern Med 2003;163(3):286–92.
4. Farrell RJ, Kelly CP. Celiac Sprue. N Eng J Med 2002;346:180–188.

of the small intestine should form the basis of a reliable diagnosis of celiac disease. Otherwise, the necessary indications for a lifelong, strict, gluten-free diet will only be obscured.

The recent remarkable increases in education and awareness of celiac disease have delighted many patients and caregivers alike. Gluten-free food aisles have appeared in some supermarkets; gluten-free menus are proudly presented by a few innovative restaurants; a US Federal standard for gluten-free food labeling is about to be introduced; the ranks of local and national celiac support groups are swelling; primary care providers are increasingly using celiac autoantibody blood tests to identify the disease in their patients, and specialized celiac centers have been established at a small number of leading medical centers across the country. However, a great deal of work remains to reverse decades of ignorance and neglect.

There is no doubt that the general US medical community remains poorly versed on the clinical presentations, diagnosis and management of celiac disease. Despite the excellent efforts of celiac advocacy groups, medical educators and the NIH Celiac Awareness campaign it will be many years before knowledge of celiac disease rises to the same level in the minds of healthcare providers as that of other similarly common and chronic medical conditions.

It is against this background that the value of Dr Burns' writings are best appreciated. More and more Americans are being diagnosed with celiac disease but are often disappointed by the dearth of information available from their regular healthcare providers about the disease, its causes, associations and treatment. This void is elegantly filled by Dr Burns' work that provides easy access to a wealth of accurate, relevant, and clearly presented information. This is especially important to those with celiac disease because the treatment, a strict gluten-free diet, demands substantial knowledge, dedication and effort. Gluten is abundant and ubiquitous in our foodstuffs and negotiating a gluten-free path requires both motivation and understanding. Individuals with celiac disease who are knowledgeable about the disorder are certainly in a better position to successfully adhere to a gluten-free diet. They are also in a better position to act as an effective advocate by supporting companies that provide easy access to gluten-free foodstuffs and by challenging those that do not.

The format chosen by Dr Burns is ideal for a readership that may have little or no previous experience with medical writings but are eager to learn more about a disorder that has changed their everyday lives in such a basic way. The book can be read from front-to-back following the logical order of its sections to obtain a comprehensive overview of this complex disease and its many manifestations. Alternatively, it can be enjoyed piecemeal by jumping to those topics and questions of most immediate interest and saving other topics for another time. I suspect most readers will use the book in both ways—sometimes reading in sequence and sometimes referring to specific sections to answer their immediate questions and those of their family and friends.

However it is used *100 Questions & Answers About Celiac Disease and Sprue* will be a valued addition to the library of anyone who lives with celiac disease or lives beside a relative or friend who must live gluten-free. It will also be extremely valuable to primary care physicians, gastroenterologists and dieticians. Those of us who are healthcare providers can always benefit from additional education on celiac disease, especially in a format that will enable us to more clearly convey that information to our patients.

Ciarán P Kelly, MD
Associate Professor of Medicine, Harvard Medical School
Director, Celiac Center, Beth Israel Deaconess Medical Center
Boston, MA

PREFACE

Roughly 1 in 100 Americans—that's approximately 3 million people—have celiac disease. Celiac disease may present with typical gastrointestinal symptoms of diarrhea, bloating, and weight loss. Celiac disease may also present atypically, manifesting as short stature in adolescents or infertility in women of childbearing age. Given the many presentations of celiac disease, including asymptomatic (no symptoms), it is a great masquerader of disease. This masquerade frequently results in a delay—an average wait of 8 years—for correct diagnosis.

I wrote this book for several reasons. Celiac disease is common, and I see patients with it on a daily basis. Most authors of books on celiac disease are patients, doctors, or dietitians. I am a subspecialist gastroenterologist who treats small intestinal diseases, malnutrition, and diseases of impaired nutrient absorption. I have training in gastroenterology and additional training in nutritional diseases and treatment. This allows me to see celiac disease from two different perspectives, which makes this book different. Because of my background, this book is weighted toward medical issues: It is a medical reference book to guide readers through the entire spectrum of celiac disease diagnosis, management, complications, disease associations and treatment, the gluten-free diet, and its drawbacks.

My first book with Jones and Bartlett Publishers was *100 Questions & Answers About Gastroesophageal Reflux Disease, A Lahey Clinic Guide.* Early into the project I realized that if you have heartburn you take an antacid or medicine that blocks acid production, but, what do you do if you have celiac disease? There is no magic pill that makes the symptoms or disease go away. You have to learn a whole new diet and way of eating that affects your entire life. The key to living with celiac disease is knowledge and education. That is the main reason I wrote this book: to teach my patients.

Patients need advice and information about managing a disease with ongoing or new symptoms, or the development of an associated complication or disease. Clinicians need to know the diseases that can mimic or exacerbate celiac disease, like lactose intolerance or microscopic colitis.

Doctors, healthcare providers, and patients need to know the associated diseases that possibly make celiac disease more likely, such as autoimmune disease like dermatitis herpetiformis. Likewise, they need to understand the increased risks of other problems, like liver or thyroid, for a patient with celiac disease. Doctors and healthcare providers need to know the way to make an appropriate diagnosis of celiac disease given different disease severities and manifestations. Patients and caregivers have to know the risks and benefits of a gluten-free diet and when it is appropriate to prescribe one.

Patients should understand the pitfalls associated with negotiating the minefield that is a gluten-free diet. Most importantly, patients with celiac disease have to learn the diet with the aid of a dietitian and other available resources. The gluten-free diet requires adequate follow-up to ensure that weight issues and/or vitamin deficiencies do not occur.

I am not a dietitian. The gluten-free diet has been well covered in other books, and for adequate discussion, it really requires hundreds of pages, which is beyond the scope of this book. Rather, I wanted to write a book that addressed all the medical issues and covered the role of a gluten-free diet, sources of gluten contamination, and resources for "where to go next."

I am not a pediatrician, and I do not treat children. Likewise, I am not a dermatologist and generally do not treat skin conditions. The information provided in this book is the most up-to-date available from the medical literature. My discussion and recommendations for children and diseases of the skin like dermatitis herpetiformis are from major medical societies that make practice guidelines for doctors. I recommend readers check with their child's pediatrician if they have questions or issues.

A number of resources were available to me in writing this book, and these are summarized in the appendix section. The most valuable resource was the Internet and my "research assistant" *Google*. The ability to get instant information on anything at any time of the day or night is incredible. This information included the latest medical articles, downloadable lists of safe foods or medications, gluten-free restaurant menus, and where to get a low-gluten host for communion. I encourage readers to use this book in conjunction with the Web to explore the provided links as further resources.

ACKNOWLEDGMENTS

Many people were involved in the production of this book. First and foremost I would like to thank the production team at Jones and Bartlett Publishers. This is my second book with Jones and Bartlett, and it was during production of my first book, *100 Questions & Answers About Gastroesophageal Reflux Disease (GERD): A Lahey Clinic Guide*, that the inspiration for this book arose. My idea for a book on celiac disease was quickly accepted by Jones and Bartlett Executive Publisher Christopher Davis, despite the fact that at the time I had not even finished my first book. But, Chris had faith in me and my ability to produce two book manuscripts.

I would also like to thank Associate Editor Kathy Richardson and Associate Production Editor Rachel Rossi for the time-consuming work of putting all the pieces together and bringing both of my books to life.

I would like to thank my patient Marye Ruzilla on her contribution to this project and her unique perspective on celiac disease, which she has to deal with on a daily basis.

I would also like to acknowledge and thank those at Lahey Clinic that contributed to the book. Mr. Rick Chevalier of medical photography prepared several photographs for the manuscript, Dr. Bruce Tronic of the Department of Pathology photographed the microscopic images of the small intestine, and Dr. Francis Scholz of the Department of Radiology provided the x-ray images.

Finally, I would like to thank my patients; you were the inspiration for this book. Education is mandatory for living with celiac disease; there is no pill or drug that is going to treat this. I wrote this book as a contribution to the educational process in understanding celiac disease and its many facets.

This book is dedicated to my family, who has supported me through the years of medical school and many subsequent years of training and work. My parents, Hedy and Arthur Burns, have been there through it all.

I am also grateful and thankful to my wife Dr. Margo Moskos and our children Stacy and Alex. Margo's patience and understanding during this project was limitless and served as an inspiration to me.

PART ONE

The Basics

What is celiac disease?

Does celiac disease run in families?

Does celiac disease affect both genders?

More...

1. What is celiac disease?

Celiac disease (CD)

Same as sprue or celiac sprue and gluten-sensitive enteropathy. A food allergy to gluten, which is a protein found in the grains wheat, barley, rye, and possibly oats. An autoimmune disease characterized by inflammation and damage to the small intestine, with resulting malabsorption of nutrients.

Small intestine

The site of digestion and absorption of nutrients.

Digestion

The process of breaking food down into simple sugars, triglycerides, and amino acids. Digestion occurs prior to absorption.

Protein

A nitrogen-containing substance that is made up of amino acids.

Amino acids

The building blocks for proteins. Dietary proteins are broken down into amino acids during the digestion process to allow for their absorption.

Celiac disease (CD) is a food allergy that primarily affects the digestive system but can also involve virtually any organ. Inflammation of and damage to the **small intestine** causes impaired absorption of the vitamins, minerals, and nutrients found in food. The small intestine is the major site for the breakdown of food, a process that involves both digestion and absorption:

- **Digestion** is the process of breaking down food into usable parts, such as the conversion of a piece of steak into **proteins** or its building blocks, **amino acids.**
- **Absorption** is the movement of these nutrients into the body for further use.

The small intestine is lined by tiny finger-like projections called the **villi** (Figure 1). The villi are where digestion and absorption of nutrients take place.

Celiac disease is an allergy to a protein called **gluten** that results in chronic inflammation and damage to the villi, which in turn interferes in the normal processing of food. Gluten is found in grains such as wheat, **rye,** and **barley.** This protein is extremely common in the human diet—for example, it makes bread dough sticky and is used as the lickable adhesive on envelopes. In celiac disease, the immune system becomes overactive and attacks itself (that is, it damages the small intestine). For this reason, this kind of disorder is called an **autoimmune disease.** In short, celiac disease causes the body to react to gluten consumed in the diet by attacking and damaging the villi, resulting in chronic inflammation and impaired absorption or **malabsorption** of nutrients.

In adults, the typical symptoms of CD include bloating, diarrhea, weight loss, and abdominal discomfort or cramps. In some cases, CD can have a variety of nonspecific symptoms that can make the diagnosis difficult, often delaying this disease's identification for many years. Children may experience

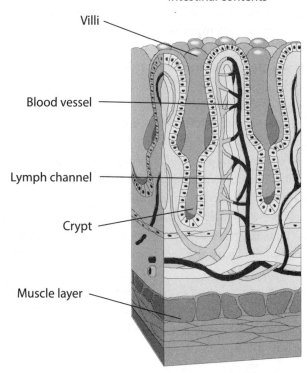

Intestinal contents

Villi

Blood vessel

Lymph channel

Crypt

Muscle layer

External intestinal surface

Figure 1   A cross section of the duodenum. The villi are the finger-like projections.

the same symptoms as adults plus poor growth, inability to gain weight, and bad teeth. Other problems that may affect both adults and children include anemia (low blood), vitamin and mineral deficiencies, and thin bones. Celiac disease is a **genetic disorder,** so it tends to run in families and in certain ethnic groups.

Unfortunately, there is no medication or real treatment for celiac disease other than the elimination of gluten-containing products from the diet. Maintaining a gluten-free diet allows the inflammation and damage to the small intestine to heal and improves the body's processing of nutrients.

The Basics

Absorption

The ability to move nutrients in the intestinal contents through the gut lining and into the bloodstream.

Villi

The finger-like projections that line the small intestine and are the sites of digestion and absorption of food.

Gluten

A protein found in wheat, rye, and barley that makes dough sticky and gooey.

Rye

A gluten-containing grain.

Barley

A gluten-containing grain.

Autoimmune disease

A type of disease in which the body attacks itself, causing damage. Examples include vitiligo, rheumatoid arthritis, lupus, and auto-immune hepatitis.

Malabsorption

The impaired absorption of consumed nutrients.

Genetic disorder

A disorder or disease passed from parent to child through the genes.

Sprue

Another name for celiac disease.

Celiac sprue

Another term for celiac disease, sprue, or gluten-sensitive enteropathy.

Non-tropical sprue

Another name for celiac disease.

Gluten-sensitive enteropathy

Another name for celiac disease.

Celiac disease goes by several names that are used interchangeably: **sprue, celiac sprue, non-tropical sprue,** and **gluten-sensitive enteropathy.**

Marye was diagnosed with celiac disease when she was 70 years old:

Before I was diagnosed with celiac disease, I had read about the silent disease in a magazine article, but did not know anyone who had it. Our local paper had recently published a story about a young girl of the Catholic faith who has celiac disease. Her mother had asked their area bishop to use a wheat substitute for the host, but the bishop denied their request. The story went on to relate the difficult time the girl was having with wheat products and the Catholic position on using a wheat substitute for the host.

[Since my diagnosis,] items I never thought of as containing gluten—such as cosmetic products, vitamins, the glue on the backs of stamps and envelopes, and prescriptions— I now double-check. I question everything.

On the positive side, many companies that I have called to ask whether their products contain gluten have sent me a list of their gluten-free products or coupons good for their products. A few have even sent free products.

2. Is celiac disease something new?

Celiac disease is not a new disease. Owing to our improved understanding of CD and more frequent testing for this condition by doctors, however, more people are now being diagnosed with it.

A disease resembling CD was first described in Turkey in the second century A.D. by Aretaeus. In more modern times, CD and its treatment with a gluten-free diet were first characterized by a Dutch pediatrician named Willem Dicke during World War II. During the 1940s, the Netherlands suffered a shortage of grains, and bread and cereal were scarce. Dicke observed that during this period fewer cases of sprue (a disease of diarrhea and weight loss) arose, and those children with sprue improved and gained weight. Once the shortage of grains resolved, the Dutch children became sick again. This phenomenon led to the discovery that the toxic agent affecting these children was something in the wheat products—namely, gluten.

In the years immediately following World War II, the diagnosis of celiac disease was based on the patient's symptoms or on a **biopsy** of the small intestine, which at the time required an operation. Over the past 20 years, however, biopsy of the small intestine has become easier thanks to the routine use of **endoscopy**, which revolutionized diagnosis of CD. Also, blood testing for CD has come into common use. This evolution in diagnostic techniques has been accompanied by increased awareness of CD among medical professionals, prompting even more testing. Celiac disease is frequently mentioned in the press, thus patient awareness has also increased, so that patients now commonly request testing for this condition. As a result of all these factors, there has been an explosion in the number of people who are diagnosed with CD and our understanding of how truly widespread CD is.

3. Is celiac disease common, and does it occur in certain ethnic groups or nationalities?

Celiac disease primarily affects people of white Northern European ancestry. In mass-population screenings conducted through blood testing, high rates of CD have been observed in parts of Italy, Canada, Ireland, Sweden, Finland, and India.

Irish people—and particularly those from County Cork and County Galway—have very high observed rates of CD. Likewise, French Canadians have high rates of the disease. In large studies done in the United States, 0.5 to 1 percent of the population tested positive for CD. Of course, the United

The Basics

Biopsy
A procedure in which the physician takes a small piece of tissue from the body for later examination under the microscope.

Endoscopy
A medical procedure in which the patient swallows a scope, allowing for examination of the gut and the opportunity to take biopsies.

Table 1   Incidence of Celiac Disease in Large Population Screenings

Group Studied	Rate of Celiac Disease
Swedish Blood Donors	1 in 256
Canadians	1 in 200
Italian School Children	1 in 184
Belfast, Ireland Adults	1 in 152
Finnish Students	1 in 99
Italian School Children*	1 in 96

* Different study

States is a "melting pot" of émigrés from other countries. Also, these tests identify "all comers," including asymptomatic people and not necessarily individuals whose family members have CD. Certainly, in selected populations the rates can be much higher.

Celiac disease is much rarer in other non-Caucasian ethnic groups. Nevertheless, it has been reported in Sudanese, Cantonese, Hispanic, Israeli Jew, and Arab populations.

4. Does celiac disease run in families?

The rates of CD among relatives of individuals with known CD vary widely. This discrepancy arises because different types of tests are used to define what CD is in different studies. Blood testing is easy and relatively cheap, and most people will allow a blood test; hence it is a good option when trying to determine CD rates in large populations. But not all of the blood tests are equivalent, and their results can vary. The "gold standard" for diagnosis is an endoscopy test with a **small intestine biopsy**—a procedure that would be difficult to use when screening a large population for the disease.

When assessed via biopsy, the rate of CD found in **first-degree relatives** of patients with proven CD ranges from 5.5 percent

Small intestine biopsy

A biopsy taken at the time of endoscopy for the purpose of making the diagnosis of celiac disease.

First-degree relative

A very closely related family member, such as a parent, a child, or a sibling.

Table 2   The Rate of Celiac Disease in Relatives of U.S. CD Patients

Group	Rate of Celiac Disease
First-Degree Relatives	1 in 22
Second-Degree Relatives	1 in 39
Symptomatic Patients	1 in 56
Not-at-risk Group	1 in 133

Adapted from Fasano et al. Arch Int Med 2003.

to 22.5 percent. Studies on second-degree relatives of patients with proven CD suggest a rate of CD that ranges from 2.6 percent to 5.5 percent. If more than one family member has CD, the rates tend to be even higher. All of these rates exceed the "baseline" rate for the average U.S. population, which is about 1 in 100 (or 1 percent). Most studies suggest that if one family member has CD, his or her first- and second-degree relatives have about a 10 percent chance of testing positive for the disease.

Celiac disease is a genetic disease that may be passed among families. Humans inherit one set of genes from each parent. Celiac disease is associated with two genes, **HLA-DQ2** and **HLA-DQ8**. To have CD, you must inherit either or both of these genes from your parents (see Question 43). Interestingly, the risk of CD is extremely high among sets of identical twins if one twin has CD. This inheritance pattern explains why CD is so common among family members.

Marye comments:

I am of Irish/German background. My mother is 103 years old and on no medication. My father was close to his 103rd birthday when he died from cancer. Over the years, Dad did have some stomach problems and was treated for a bleeding ulcer. Mom was always in good health.

If one family member has CD, his or her first- and second-degree relatives have about a 10 percent chance of testing positive for the disease.

HLA-DQ2/HLA-DQ8

The two genes that predispose a person to having celiac disease.

The Basics

7

After I was diagnosed with celiac disease, I questioned both my maternal and paternal relatives about whether they had any allergies to food. I found out that one relative was allergic to milk in any form, and both she and her daughter had problems with their bones breaking. Several cousins have had different stomach problems such as Crohn's disease.

5. Does celiac disease affect both genders?

Several large studies of patients with CD demonstrate a female-to-male patient ratio of 1.5–2:1. However, this ratio may not be entirely trustworthy. Celiac disease commonly causes poor absorption of dietary **iron,** resulting in anemia or low blood cell counts. This effect can be aggravated in women, because they have a higher risk of anemia related to the blood and iron losses produced by the menstrual cycle. These factors favor the evaluation of anemia in women, which may in turn prompt more testing for and more frequent diagnosis of CD. Similarly, osteoporosis (thinning of the bones) is more common in women and may prompt testing for CD. The female-to-male ratio may also be biased by the fact that women generally seek medical attention more often than men and, therefore, are more likely to be tested for CD. All of these factors may act together to increase the rate at which CD is diagnosed in women.

Smaller studies suggest a female-to-male patient ratio that is closer to 1:1, and clinical experience confirms this finding. Overall, women may be diagnosed with CD more often, but female sex in general does not necessarily predispose you to CD.

6. Are celiac disease, celiac sprue, and sprue the same thing? And what about tropical sprue and gluten sensitivity?

Celiac disease goes by several names, which are used interchangeably by both the general population and health pro-

Iron

A mineral stored in the body that is used to make hemoglobin, the protein that carries oxygen. Low iron levels can cause anemia.

fessionals. Whatever the name used—celiac disease, celiac sprue, sprue, non-tropical sprue, or gluten-sensitive enteropathy—the disease remains the same.

Some other diseases have similar names but are not equivalent to CD, however. **Tropical sprue,** for example, closely resembles CD but is actually a different disease entity. Its symptoms include diarrhea, cramps, and weight loss, accompanied by anemia and vitamin deficiencies. Tropical sprue occurs in warm climates such as Puerto Rico, the Dominican Republic, Cuba, India, and Southeast Asia. This infectious disease affects the small intestine, and the results of a small intestine biopsy will be similar to those seen with CD. Although the infectious agent has not been identified, tropical sprue is treatable with a course of antibiotics given over six months.

Some people can have a **gluten sensitivity** yet not have CD. These patients experience symptoms when they consume gluten but test negative for CD. Gluten sensitivity is not an allergy, and small intestine biopsies will be normal in such cases. Gluten is a difficult protein to digest, and its processing requires a lot of coordinated work by the small intestine, stomach, and pancreas. Many patients with irritable bowel syndrome (IBS) have gluten sensitivity, for example: They develop cramps, bloating, and diarrhea after eating gluten. Such symptoms are usually treated by switching to a gluten-free or low-gluten diet. Because individuals with gluten sensitivity do not experience inflammation of and damage to the small intestine, they should not have weight loss or any vitamin deficiencies.

7. Is celiac disease related to other food allergies?

The short answer is no. People with CD may have sensitivities to other foods, and physicians may suggest removing or restricting eating certain foods from the diet.

Tropical sprue
An infectious disease of the small intestine that mimics celiac disease and is treated with antibiotics.

Gluten sensitivity
A food sensitivity to gluten that causes symptoms but is not an allergy. In such a patient, testing will be negative for celiac disease.

The Basics

Lactose

A sugar in cow's milk that can cause symptoms for those individuals with lactose intolerance.

Enzymes

Proteins produced in the pancreas that break down food to its simplest type of nutrient for subsequent absorption.

Lactose intolerance

A common disorder characterized by the loss of the ability to digest lactose. Symptoms include cramps, diarrhea, and gas.

Lactase

An enzyme produced in the small intestine that digests the sugar lactose found in cow's milk.

Low-residue diet

A diet with a roughage restriction.

In particular, dairy products should be avoided (at least early after a diagnosis of CD). Milk contains a sugar called **lactose** that is broken down or digested in the small intestine by **enzymes** on the villi. In CD, the villi are inflamed and do not function well. One of the first manifestations of this problem is the loss of the body's ability to digest lactose, a condition called **lactose intolerance.** Lactose intolerance (which is not an allergy) is characterized by development of diarrhea, gas, bloating, and/or cramps after having milk products. Lactose intolerance is very common and many people lose the ability to digest milk as they age, particularly within certain ethnic groups. Eastern European Jews, African Americans, Chinese, and Hispanic adults are often lactose intolerant. Unlike with CD, however, a digestive enzyme (called **lactase**) is available to help digest lactose and improve affected individuals' symptoms. A variety of pills and predigested bottled milk containing lactase are widely available in most supermarkets.

When patients stick to a gluten-free diet, after a few months the damage heals and their ability to digest lactose may return. In such cases, milk products can be reintroduced into the diet to see if they cause symptoms. In addition, if you are uncertain about your ability to digest lactose, your doctor can order simple tests to check for lactose intolerance.

For people with severe CD who experience a large weight loss and frequent diarrhea, their physicians may recommend a low-fiber or **low-residue diet.** This kind of diet is easier to digest and may improve some individuals' symptoms. In a low-residue diet, roughage—that is, most raw fruits, vegetable, and foods high in fiber—is avoided or limited.

Examples of lactose-free or low-residue diets are available from your doctor, from a dietitian, or on the Internet. My general recommendation to patients who have recently been diagnosed with CD is, in addition to following a gluten-free diet, to initially consume a lactose-free diet. For those who are very symptomatic with severe diarrhea, I might add a recommendation of a low-residue diet. Unfortunately, this set of recommendations does not leave much to eat, so many patients complain about its limitations. In my practice, I try to reintroduce foods as quickly as possible in such cases. Luckily, once patients have been gluten free for a while, consumption of many items can be resumed.

Another common food allergy is sensitivity to nuts; this allergy is not related to or associated with CD. Other less common food allergies focus on apples, pears, kiwis, strawberries, **soy,** and whey (a protein in milk). None of these conditions is related to CD and, in fact, they generally have different symptoms. These allergies may cause wheezing or difficulty breathing, itchiness, rash, cramps, or **anaphylaxis** (a life-threatening allergic reaction). None of these food allergies produce the inflammation of and damage to the small intestine like that seen in CD.

The Basics

Soy

A gluten-free starch. It is *not* equivalent to soy sauce.

Anaphylaxis

A severe, life-threatening allergic reaction that can be fatal.

PART TWO

Symptoms and Manifestations

Are there different kinds of celiac disease?

Can I have celiac disease without any symptoms?

What is the association between lactose intolerance and celiac disease?

More . . .

8. What are the typical gastrointestinal symptoms of celiac disease?

Celiac disease has many different manifestations and frequently masquerades as other diseases, which sometimes makes its diagnosis difficult. Its severity can fall anywhere along a spectrum ranging from completely asymptomatic to mild symptoms to life-threatening disease resulting in death. Thankfully, most patients have mild disease and death is a rarity. Most commonly, patients experience diarrhea, vomiting, cramps, abdominal pain, and either weight loss or the inability to gain weight. Adult patients frequently report that they have a lifelong history of stomach problems and were always on the thin side.

Many people with CD have increased gas, bloating, cramps, and large, bulky, foul-smelling stools. These problems arise when undigested food moves through the gut to the colon, which is full of beneficial bacteria that aid in the digestive process. These bacteria produce gas and other by-products that result in the symptoms. The small intestine, which is the organ of digestion and absorption of nutrients, acts as a barrier to this process. It serves as a gatekeeper that does not allow the movement of some toxins or bacteria from the gut into the body (or vice versa) and keeps fluids, proteins, and vital salts in the body from leaking out. Common gastrointestinal (GI) symptoms of CD are related to the damage inflicted on this area and the small intestine's inability to do its normal job. When a person has CD, his or her stools may be foul smelling, be gray or pale, float, be greasy or have an oil slick, or be frothy or gassy. Incontinence of stool can be very distressing for patients, affecting their lifestyles. Some may prefer not to leave home because of this issue, eventually becoming housebound. If the damage to the small intestine is severe, then the symptoms can also be severe, including life-threatening weight loss and diarrhea.

Weight loss in CD is related to improper absorption of nutrients. It is similar to continually dieting in that 100 percent of ingested food is not appropriately processed. However, being obese or overweight does not eliminate or exclude the diagnosis of CD. Malabsorption of nutrients can lead to vitamin and mineral deficiencies such as anemia, osteoporosis, and vitamin B_{12} deficiency.

Vitamin B_{12}
A vitamin required for blood production and nerve and brain function. A deficiency of B_{12} can require monthly vitamin shots.

Table 3   Symptoms Associated with Celiac Disease

Gastrointestinal Symptoms
  Gas and bloating
  Abdominal pain
  Chronic diarrhea
  Pale, bulky, foul-smelling stools

Systemic Symptoms
  Weight loss
  Recurrent dehydration
  Fatigue
  Muscle weakness or cramps
  Seizures
  Bone pain
  Arthritis
  Numbness or tingling in arms or legs
  Missed or irregular periods
  Infertility and recurrent miscarriages
  Delayed growth or short stature
  Mouth ulcers
  Tooth discoloration with enamel loss
  Hair and nail changes
  Rash, dermatitis herpetiformis
  Psychiatric illness
  Anemia or iron deficiency
  Osteoporosis or vitamin D deficiency

Symptoms in children may differ from those seen in adults. In particular, young children with CD may have failure to thrive, accompanied by weight loss, inability to gain weight, and failure to grow normally. They may feed poorly and be colicky. Diarrhea can be of variable severity but present at any age. Short stature and dental problems are associated with undiagnosed CD from childhood.

Marye comments:

My gastrointestinal symptoms included diarrhea that would start within one-half hour after I ate a meal. Once I started the gluten-free diet, I noticed that the pains in my hands and feet had diminished, and I was not as tired as I had been. I also found that I had diarrhea only when I ate something in error.

9. What are non-intestinal symptoms or systemic manifestations of celiac disease?

When patients with CD have symptoms, they may be so varied that the diagnosis is missed or delayed by years. The average patient with CD waits eight years before his or her disease is diagnosed.

Celiac disease is frequently asymptomatic—that is, affected individuals may have no symptoms at all. When patients do have symptoms, they may be so varied that the diagnosis is missed or delayed by years. Indeed, the average patient with CD waits eight years before his or her disease is diagnosed. It is hoped that in the future, the greater ease in testing for CD provided by the introduction of blood tests and the increased patient and doctor awareness will lead to shorter gaps between the development of symptoms and the definitive diagnosis of CD. Patient education through the Internet and medical websites where patients can plug in their symptoms and various diagnoses are suggested can help to narrow the possible causes of the patient's symptoms. Today, many patients research their symptoms online and ask their doctors to check them for CD.

Symptoms can be broken down into several categories: none or asymptomatic, gastrointestinal symptoms, or systemic/non-GI symptoms. Many new patients diagnosed with CD have few or no symptoms and are referred for treatment because of **anemia**. Routine blood tests may show a low **hematocrit (HCT)** or **hemoglobin (Hb)** level, which leads to the diagnosis of anemia. Iron from the diet is required for production of red blood cells, which function to carry oxygen. In CD, the area of the small intestine that normally takes up iron is damaged; iron is therefore poorly absorbed, resulting in anemia. Anemia is the most common blood test abnormality seen

Anemia

A low blood cell count or level, which has many causes.

Hematocrit (HCT)

A blood test for anemia.

Hemoglobin (Hb)

A blood test for anemia.

Table 4   The Spectrum of Multisystem Disease Associated with Gluten Allergy

General	Brain
Impaired Growth	Depression
Increased cancer risk	Seizures
Anemia	Ataxia
Weight loss	Numbness and tingling
Vitamin deficiency	
Iron deficiency	
Muscle cramps and weakness	
Gastrointestinal	**Mouth**
Diarrhea	Recurrent oral ulcers
Abdominal pain	Dental enamel loss
Gas and Bloating	Tongue changes
Malnutrition	
Liver abnormalities	
Weight loss	
Skin	**Bone**
Dermatitis herpetiformis	Osteoporosis
Vitiligo	Osteopenia
Eczema	Fractures
Reproductive	**Endocrine**
Delayed puberty	Thyroid abnormalities
Infertility	Diabetes
Recurrent miscarriage	

in CD. Checking for CD is part of the medical evaluation carried out when a person has unexplained anemia. Commonly, young women are anemic, a condition that is often dismissed as menstrual-related blood loss. Such women should be treated with iron supplements. If their anemia does not improve with this treatment or if they have a family history of CD, these patients should undergo testing for CD.

Anemia is the most common blood test abnormality seen in CD.

Another group of patients who may be asymptomatic for CD are those diagnosed with thinning of the bones, a condition called **osteoporosis.** Routine care after age 50 should include periodic testing for bone density, which is a diagnostic tool for detection of osteoporosis. In other cases, the diagnosis of osteoporosis is made after an unexpected bone fracture, such as breaking a toe after bumping into a piece of furniture. When it occurs in conjunction with CD, osteoporosis is caused by

Osteoporosis
Severe thinning of the bone with increased risk of fractures.

Vitamin D

A fat-soluble vitamin found in dairy products that maintains bone health.

Eczema

A scaly, itchy red rash that is associated with autoimmune disease.

Dermatitis herpetiformis (DH)

An intensely itchy rash with tiny blisters that occurs on the elbows, wrists, shoulders, and back. Virtually all patients with DH have celiac disease and should go on a gluten-free diet.

Dental enamel

The white hard covering on teeth. Abnormal dental enamel in children can be a sign of celiac disease.

Aphthous stomatitis

See *Aphthous mouth ulcers* in the glossary (p. 195).

inadequate absorption of dietary calcium and **vitamin D** over many years. Blood levels of vitamin D and calcium are low in such patients but can be corrected with calcium and vitamin D supplements. Doctors may screen for CD when patients are newly diagnosed with osteoporosis.

Rashes are often associated with CD. Both children and adults may have **eczema,** which is characterized by itchy, scaly skin. A rash that is closely associated with CD is **dermatitis herpetiformis (DH).** This intensely itchy rash features tiny blisters that cluster on the arms, legs, back, and chest. Dermatitis herpetiformis is difficult to diagnose because patients frequently scratch the rash; as a result, the blisters may be gone by the time they visit the doctor's office. Biopsy of the skin is required to diagnose DH, as microscopic skin changes may be present. In this quick and simple procedure, a small piece of skin is removed and then analyzed under a microscope.

Oral manifestations of CD may include discolored teeth from the loss of **dental enamel** (the white covering on the teeth). Recurrent mouth ulcers or sores known as **aphthous stomatitis** are also common in CD. Various vitamin and mineral deficiencies can cause skin breakdown, leading to ulceration at the corners of the lips. Tongue changes may include loss of the normal bumpy surface of the tongue, so that it has a flat, shiny appearance. Any of these changes should prompt a check for CD.

More generalized, nonspecific symptoms of CD include fatigue, depression, malaise, and lassitude. In teenagers, puberty can be delayed. Likewise, fertility problems are not uncommon in CD. Women may have difficulty becoming pregnant and, once pregnant, spontaneous losses of the pregnancy are common during the first trimester (that is, the first 12 weeks after conception).

Psychiatric and neurological problems associated with CD include depression, anxiety, irritability, seizures, numbness or tingling of the arms and legs, difficulty seeing at night, and migraines, to name a few. Muscle abnormalities are common and include recurrent muscle cramps, wasting or thinning, and weakness resulting in falls or difficulty standing and walking. In addition to osteoporosis, patients may experience bone pain (aching bones). Arthritis, which consists of inflammation and pain in the joints such as the hips and knees, affects approximately 25 percent of all people with CD.

Because abnormal absorption of nutrients is altered in CD, patients may develop "protein-calorie malnutrition." This problem can impair the body's ability to heal wounds or fight off infections. In addition, **malnutrition** affects vitamin metabolism and can result in a variety of vitamin deficiencies.

10. Are there different kinds of celiac disease?

Several types of CD are distinguished, but all are forms of the same disease. The various classifications are generally made based on the presence and type of symptoms. Other classifications of CD are based on the degree of inflammation on biopsy. Interestingly enough, the severity of symptoms may not correlate with the amount of inflammation.

Classic CD manifests as atrophy of the villi, malabsorption with vitamin deficiencies or fatty stools, and improvement of these problems after gluten is removed from the diet. Several variations on these three criteria are used to distinguish the type of CD, but their use is mostly a matter of semantics. The treatment—switching to a gluten-free diet—is the same in any event. In my practice, I generally do not use these alternative classifications because they are confusing and do not really change the outcome.

Atypical CD is probably the most common manifestation of sprue. These patients do not have any gastrointestinal symptoms but may demonstrate infertility, anemia, or osteoporosis. These patients come to their doctors complaining of non-

Malnutrition

A disease of inadequate nutrition, caused by either lack of access to food or impaired food absorption.

Classic celiac disease

Celiac disease that presents with symptoms of diarrhea, weight loss, and bloating.

Atypical celiac disease

Celiac disease that manifests without typical symptoms.

intestinal symptoms, only to ultimately be diagnosed with CD.

Undiagnosed celiac disease

The presence of symptoms without a diagnosis that is eventually recognized as celiac disease.

In **undiagnosed CD,** the patient has the typical symptoms and inflammation of the villi, but confirmatory blood tests for CD have not been done yet. Although inflammation and shortening of the villi are the hallmarks of CD, they are nonspecific findings on biopsy and can be present in other conditions. Consequently, blood tests are required to support the definitive diagnosis of CD.

Silent celiac disease

Asymptomatic celiac disease.

Latent celiac disease

An asymptomatic type of celiac disease in which the patient generally has a normal small intestinal biopsy.

Silent CD is the absence of symptoms in an individual who has a positive small bowel biopsy and positive celiac blood tests. In **latent or potential CD,** the person may have had CD as a child but his or her symptoms have gone away despite resumption of a gluten-containing diet; alternatively, the patient may have had normal biopsies but developed CD at a later age. Although there is some debate in the literature on this point, generally most experts do not recommend a gluten-free diet for patients with latent or potential CD.

Once the diagnosis of CD is established, the individual's response to a gluten-free diet can change the type of CD he or she is considered to have. Classification into one of these categories has greater medical significance than the type of CD identified on initial diagnosis, as it affects treatment plans and patient outcomes. Many patients with CD become symptomatic again despite faithfully following a gluten-free diet. In some cases, the problem stems from unknown gluten contaminating the diet, a phenomenon known as **surreptitious gluten ingestion.** It can be sorted out by repeating the blood testing for CD. If the test is positive, then there is gluten in the diet; if it is negative, then gluten is not the cause.

Surreptitious gluten ingestion

Ingestion of gluten from an unknown source.

When symptoms recur despite consumption of a gluten-free diet, patients should be sent back to the dietitian to have their diet reviewed. If no gluten is found, then the patient likely has

refractory sprue (also known as **refractory CD**). This group of patients includes those with classic CD that either never responded to a gluten-free diet or did respond only to have symptoms recur. Refractory sprue is a serious condition that can result in severe malabsorption and death; its treatment may require medications that suppress the immune system, such as steroids. A subset of those patients with refractory sprue have scarring or increased fibrosis of the small intestine on biopsy, a condition called **collagenous sprue**.

11. Can I have celiac disease without any symptoms?

Although CD usually has symptoms, it is occasionally diagnosed in people without any physical symptoms. This frequently happens when first-degree relatives of patients with CD are screened, such as a child or sibling of someone with CD. Approximately 1 in 10 (10 percent) of these first-degree relatives will test positive for CD, though these people are generally asymptomatic.

Individuals with unexplained anemia or osteoporosis may also be screened by their doctors for CD. This testing is intended to detect a cause of impaired absorption of dietary iron (in case of anemia) or vitamin D (in case of osteoporosis). Generally, individuals with these conditions do not have any physical symptoms of CD, but their disease may be discovered on blood tests or scans before they develop symptoms. In the medical literature, people who have positive blood tests for CD but no symptoms are said to have "subclinical disease." Patients with latent CD and silent CD are generally asymptomatic.

12. Which other diseases are associated with celiac disease?

Celiac disease is an autoimmune disease, meaning that the body identifies part of itself as "foreign" and then attacks the

Refractory (sprue) celiac disease

Celiac disease that does not respond to a gluten-free diet.

Collagenous sprue

A type of difficult or refractory sprue that may require additional medication to suppress the immune system.

Symptoms and Manifestations

Celiac disease is an autoimmune disease, meaning that the body identifies part of itself as "foreign" and then attacks the "invader." Because of this association, many other autoimmune diseases may occur in conjunction with CD.

"invader" (that is, itself). Because of this association, many other autoimmune diseases may occur in conjunction with CD. A family history of autoimmune disease may also be present.

Table 5   Diseases Associated with Celiac Disease

Autoimmune Diseases
  Dermatitis herpetiformis
  Thyroid disease, like Grave's disease or Hashimoto's thyroiditis,
      hyperactive (over active) or hypoactive (under active) thyroid
  Type 1 or Juvenile Diabetes
  Vitiligo, loss of skin pigment with white patches on the skin
  Ezcema
  Dry mouth or Sicca syndrome
  Lupus
  Rheumatoid arthritis
  Autoimmune liver disease like primary biliary cirrhosis

Other Disease Associations
  Abnormal liver tests
  Fatty liver disease
  Anemia
  Osteoporosis
  Pernicious anemia
  Down syndrome
  Turner syndrome
  Williams syndrome
  Selective IgA deficiency
  Bacterial overgrowth
  Microscopic colitis

Celiac disease is also associated with other diseases that are not autoimmune in nature, and some of these disease associations are very strong. People with type 1 diabetes, for example, have a 3 to 10 percent chance of having CD. Individuals with Down syndrome have a 5 to 10 percent chance of developing CD. **Selective immunoglobulin A (IgA) deficiency** is a disorder of the immune system that manifests as recurrent ear infections in children, recurrent sinus infections, pneumonia, and bronchitis. Five percent of those with CD have a selective IgA deficiency, which creates difficulties in diagnosis because the blood test for CD can be falsely negative in these patients.

Selective immuno-globulin A (IgA) deficiency

The most common immunodeficiency, caused by inability to produce IgA.

Microscopic colitis is an inflammatory condition of the large intestine that is manifested as chronic watery diarrhea. Generally, the affected person does not experience any weight loss or blood in the stool. The diagnosis of microscopic colitis is made via a colonoscopy, which should look normal. Biopsies are taken during the colonoscopy and then examined under the microscope; if the person has microscopic colitis, they will show inflammation of the lining of the colon. This is a common finding in CD. When microscopic colitis is diagnosed, the patient also needs to be checked for CD, as the treatments for the two diseases are different.

Bacterial overgrowth often complicates CD. All humans normally have bacteria in the gut. These bacteria generally live peacefully in our intestines, where they help us digest food and make some vitamins. Sometimes the numbers or types of bacteria may change, leading to problems that resemble the symptoms of CD: diarrhea, weight loss, anemia, and vitamin deficiencies. Bacterial overgrowth can be treated with antibiotics.

13. Which laboratory or blood abnormalities are associated with celiac disease?

Because CD has so many different symptoms and manifestations, the blood abnormalities associated with it are also quite variable. Blood abnormalities are relevant in two ways. First, they may be a clue that leads to the diagnosis of CD. Second, they may require treatment. The diagnostic blood tests for CD are covered in Question 38.

Abnormal blood tests can be broken out into two groups: those commonly seen in CD and those related to vitamin and mineral deficiencies. The tests listed in Table 6 are not specific to CD but rather are blood abnormalities that *may* be seen in CD. Generally speaking, any of these abnormalities require further evaluation by your doctor and should not be ignored or dismissed.

Microscopic colitis
A type of inflammation of the colon that causes diarrhea and can be identified via biopsy.

Bacterial overgrowth
The normal small intestine contains small numbers of bacteria that aid in digestion and make vitamins. In bacterial overgrowth, the number and type of bacteria increase, resulting in diarrhea, weight loss, and vitamin deficiencies.

Symptoms and Manifestations

Table 6   Blood-Testing Abnormalities That May Be Associated with Celiac Disease

General
Anemia or low Hb or HCT
Increased sedimentation rate (ESR a marker for inflammation)
Increased C-reactive protein (marker for inflammation)
Increased liver tests
Low immunoglobulin A (IgA) level
Low calcium
Increased parathyroid hormone level (PTH)
Abnormal thyroid tests (high or low)
Abnormal electrolytes
Elevated blood sugar in children
Abnormal kidney function tests
Abnormal hormone levels
Abnormal appearing red blood cells

Blood Tests Suggesting Malabsorption
Low albumin (protein)
Low prealbumin (protein)
Low transferrin (protein)
Low iron level or ferritin
Low zinc level
Low carotene or vitamin A
Low vitamin B_{12} (pernicious anemia)
Low folic acid level
Low vitamin C level (scurvy)
Low vitamin D level (osteoporosis or Rickets)
Low vitamin K level

Obesity

The condition of being overweight by about 30 pounds. Obesity increases a person's risk of cancer, stroke, diabetes, and heart disease.

Body mass index (BMI)

A measure of weight as a function of height. A BMI of less than 18 is considered underweight, 20 to 25 is normal, 25 to 30 is overweight, and greater than 30 is obese.

Marye comments:

For the antiendomysial blood test, a score of 20 or less is considered good. After three months of trying to watch what I ate, my score was 117.

14. I am overweight. How can I have celiac disease?

The U.S. population is, in general, gaining weight, and **obesity** is an increasing problem that is becoming an epidemic. The **body mass index (BMI)** is a standardized way to measure the relationship between a person's weight relative to his or her height, thereby determining whether the individual is underweight, normal weight, overweight, or obese. Many websites will calculate your BMI automatically after you enter your height and weight.

BMI Formula: English System Version
BMI = (weight in pounds) ÷ [(height in inches) × (height in inches)] × 703

BMI Formula: Metric Version
BMI = (weight in kilograms) ÷ [(height in meters) × (height in meters)]

A person is considered to be underweight if he or she has a BMI of less than 18 and to be of normal weight if he or she has a BMI in the range of 20 to 25. Overweight is defined as having a BMI between 25 and 30; obesity is defined as a BMI greater than 30. As a point of reference, if your BMI is 40 or greater, you qualify under insurance company criteria for a gastric bypass procedure. A person with a BMI of 30 is roughly 30 pounds overweight.

As can be seen in Figure 2 (which is adapted from data published by the National Institutes for Health), two thirds of Americans (66 percent) are overweight. More sobering, one third of Americans (33 percent) are obese or severely obese (more than 100 pounds overweight). Obesity is increasing in U.S. children and adults at an alarming rate. In the mid-1970s, 10 percent of the U.S. population was classified as obese, and severe obesity was rare; today, 33 percent of Americans are obese, and 7 percent are severely obese.

Multiple factors contribute to the obesity epidemic. Notably, we have become a sedentary society: We drive from place to place rather than walking. Most of us have desk jobs and do not perform physically active labor. Our children play inside, use the computer, or play video games instead of going outside to play ball or ride a bicycle. In addition to our decreasing level of physical activity, the other major contributor to the obesity epidemic is changes in our diet. Historically, we as a society

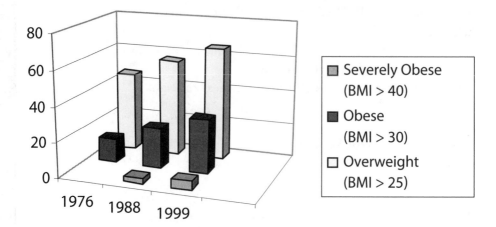

Figure 2   The epidemic of weight gain and obesity in the United States. The vertical axis depicts the percentage of the population and the horizontal axis shows the year.

used to eat at home as a family, consuming food prepared at home. Now food is available everywhere—particularly fast food, which is as plentiful as it is "supersized" and cheap. These factors have all contributed to the obesity epidemic to which we are all exposed, including people with CD.

Classically, the patient with CD, both as a child and as an adult, was underweight with a bloated abdomen and thin, spindly arms and legs—the very picture of malnutrition. To-day, however, things have changed. A recent study looked at 371 patients newly diagnosed with CD, examining their weight distribution and BMIs to determine the proportions who were underweight, normal weight, overweight, and obese. At diagnosis, 5 percent of patients were underweight, 56 percent were normal weight, and 39 percent overweight; in the last group, 13 percent of subjects were obese. This study was done over the period 1995 to 2005; when the data for 1995–2000 were compared to the data for 2001–2005, a trend toward more obesity was obvious, mirroring the findings in Figure 2.

The overall trend toward higher weights may, in turn, make diagnosis of CD more difficult. Doctors generally think of patients with CD as being thin and underweight, but today that description may fit only a small minority of patients. Ninety-five percent of celiac patients are normal or overweight.

The study mentioned earlier also provided good evidence that a person's starting weight does not predict his or her risk of developing CD. Interestingly, there was no mention of the amount of weight loss patients had experienced before their diagnosis. The same study also looked at weight trends over time after individuals had switched to a gluten-free diet. More than 80 percent of the patients on a gluten-free diet gained weight—a cause for alarm. At the start of the study, 39 percent of patients were overweight; approximately two years later, 51 percent had become overweight.

Marye comments:

I am overweight and trying to watch what I eat. I have added more fresh vegetables, fruits, and yogurt to my diet.

15. I have irritable bowel syndrome. Should I be checked for celiac disease?

Irritable bowel syndrome (IBS) is an extremely common disorder that is characterized by abdominal cramps or pain associated with altered bowel habits with constipation, diarrhea, or both, lasting more than three months. Patients may also experience bloating, excessive gas, passage of mucus, the sensation of needing to go to the bathroom urgently, or a feeling of incomplete emptying with a bowel movement.

Irritable bowel syndrome is a common reason to visit the doctor and the number one reason to visit a gastrointestinal specialist. In fact, this condition may account for 30 to 50 percent of all GI patients. The frequency with which IBS

Irritable bowel syndrome (IBS) is a common disorder that is characterized by abdominal cramps or pain associated with altered bowel habits with constipation, diarrhea, or both, lasting more than three months.

occurs makes many doctors complacent or lazy about investigating other potential causes of their patients' GI problems, or they simply may not feel that an evaluation is warranted. The symptoms associated with IBS are fairly nonspecific, so IBS often becomes a "wastebasket" diagnosis or a diagnosis of exclusion. For example, if you have cramps and altered bowel habits, your doctor may simply label it as IBS rather than doing an appropriate evaluation with blood tests, x-rays, or endoscopy tests. The average patient with IBS symptoms who actually has CD waits eight years before the correct diagnosis is made. Of note, none of the blood abnormalities mentioned earlier should be present in IBS, and blood work should be normal.

The causes of IBS are largely unknown. Given the nonspecific symptoms, this catch-all label may actually represent several different diseases that have conveniently been lumped together. The general consensus in the medical literature is that IBS is caused by an altered sensation of intestinal pain. What may be normal to the person without IBS is, instead, perceived as pain in a person with IBS.

One possible cause of this disorder is "post-infectious IBS," which typically occurs after a bout of food poisoning, a parasitic infection, or a severe diarrheal illness. In this case, the person goes on to develop altered bowel habits associated with cramps or pain. These symptoms can persist for months to years.

Metamucil

A fiber supplement used to regulate bowel movements.

Citrucil

A synthetic fiber supplement that is available over the counter.

Gluten free

A food that does not contain any gluten.

Initial treatment for IBS is a change in the diet and removal of certain foods from the diet. Restricted foods may include chocolate, dairy products and milk, fatty foods, caffeinated products, sodas, and alcohol. Some patients with CD may experience improved symptoms with these dietary changes, again reinforcing the misdiagnosis of IBS.

Adding fiber to the diet is also beneficial for treating IBS. A typical dose of a fiber supplement such as **Metamucil** or

Citrucel contains 2 to 3 grams of fiber. A bowl of high-fiber cereal may contain 6 to 10 grams of fiber. The recommended daily allotment (RDA) for fiber is 25 to 30 grams per day. Few, if any, Americans meet this recommendation, as we tend to eat more processed food that is low in fiber—and no one eats three bowls of All-Bran or takes 10 doses of Metamucil per day. Thankfully, even consuming only modest doses of fiber will help with IBS. People with CD who experience gas, bloating, and diarrhea can often benefit from these particular fiber supplements, some of which are **gluten free.**

Medications are part of the treatment regimen for IBS symptoms that cannot be controlled by diet alone. People with constipation symptoms may benefit from fiber and water in addition to laxatives and stool softeners. For example, they may gain relief with **milk of magnesia, Miralax,** or **glycolax.** Increased fluid or water consumption of eight 8-ounce glasses of water per day is beneficial. Although fiber will help patients with diarrhea, they may also need to take antidiarrheal medications such as **Imodium** or **Lomotil.** These drugs will help with his or her altered bowel habits and may improve cramps.

The gut consists of the long tube that runs from your mouth to your bottom. This tube is made up of **smooth muscle.** The smooth muscle works automatically to move food and products of digestion downstream; they are not under your conscious control. Cramps or muscle spasms of the gut may develop because of gas, bloating, diarrhea, or constipation; a variety of medications can be used to "relax" the gut. Table 7 lists some medications that are commonly used to treat muscle spasms and cramps. Many other **antispasmodic drugs** are available as well.

Interestingly, these medications frequently help for symptoms of CD, again contributing to the confusion and delay in diagnosis. This is a short list and there are many other anti-spasmotic drugs available.

Symptoms and Manifestations

Milk of magnesia
A laxative medication used to treat constipation.

Miralax
A type of laxative commonly used to prepare the bowel for a colonoscopy.

Glycolax
A type of laxative that is commonly used as preparation for a colonoscopy.

Imodium
A drug used to treat diarrhea.

Lomotil
A prescription medication used to treat diarrhea.

Smooth muscle
The muscle in the lining of the intestine that moves materials forward in the gut.

Antispasmodic drugs
A class of medications used to relax the intestines. These drugs are commonly prescribed for patients with irritable bowel syndrome. Examples include Bentyl, Levsin, and Donnatal.

Table 7   Antispasmodic Drugs Used to Treat Irritable Bowel Syndrome

Generic Name	Proprietary Name
Dicyclomine	Bentyl
Hyoscyamine	Levsin, Nulex, Levbid, Pamine
Scopolamine	Scop patch
Clidinium/Librium	Librax
Phenobarbital/Hyoscyamine/ Atropine/Scopolamine	Donnatal

The short answer to this question is all patients with IBS should be checked for CD. This eliminates the delay in diagnosis of CD and to rule out the misdiagnosis of IBS. Many celiac symptoms will resolve if the patient adheres to a gluten-free diet, thereby avoiding the need to take unnecessary medication. Individuals with IBS should have blood testing to exclude CD because some people with IBS can have improved symptoms on a gluten-free diet. These people may have a sensitivity to gluten but do not have CD or a true allergy to wheat products.

16. What is the association between lactose intolerance and celiac disease?

Lactose intolerance is a very common disorder characterized by diarrhea, gas, bloating, and possibly cramps after eating dairy products such as milk, ice cream, or cheese, or foods that contain these items. Milk from cows contains a sugar called lactose. Lactose consumed in the diet is digested or broken down on the surface of the villi of the small intestine by an enzyme called lactase. We frequently lose the ability to metabolize or digest lactose either temporarily or permanently, resulting in lactose intolerance.

Children can have lactose intolerance and need to be on a dairy product–restricted diet. Sometimes we outgrow our ability to make lactase; as we age, the production of this enzyme decreases and new symptoms develop. Once this occurs, it is generally permanent. The good news is that enzyme supplements are available to help with symptoms and digestion. Lactose intolerance is very common in certain ethnic groups—especially African Americans, Hispanics, Chinese people, and European Jews—but can occur in anyone.

There is a very close association between lactose intolerance and CD. Celiac disease involves inflammation and damage to the villi, the metabolically active site of digestion and absorption of nutrients in the small intestine. This is the same site where the lactase is produced, so one of the first results of CD-related damage to the villi is loss of lactase production. As a consequence, many patients with CD are lactose intolerant. For this reason, when I diagnose a patient with new CD in my practice, I recommend both a gluten-free and a lactose-free diet. Once the patient has been gluten free for a while, I recommend adding back the dairy products—after the damage to the small intestine has healed, lactase production may return and the lactose intolerance disappear.

Lactose intolerance can be easily diagnosed based on its symptoms. If you drink milk and get diarrhea shortly thereafter, then you likely are lactose intolerant. If there is any question, I tell my patients to avoid consuming milk, ice cream, cheese, and dairy-containing products for a week; if the symptoms go away, then they are probably lactose intolerant.

Some patients insist on being more scientific and want a test called a **lactose breath test**. This easy but time-consuming test is performed in the doctor's office. The patient drinks a lactose-containing liquid. Every 15 to 30 minutes, his or her breath is collected in a plastic bag, and the gas is then analyzed. If the patient cannot digest the lactose, it travels through the small intestine to the colon or large intestine, which is full of bacteria. These bacteria digest the lactose and produce hydrogen gas and other products, which lead to bloating and diarrhea. Some of the gas is expelled as flatus; some

Lactose breath test
A test for lactose intolerance.

is taken up through the bloodstream and exhaled from the lungs. Hydrogen is not normally produced by humans, so its presence in the breath test after lactose consumption signals that the person is lactose intolerant.

Finally, there is help for those with lactose intolerance: They do not have to completely eliminate milk and dairy products from their diet, unlike the complete avoidance of gluten that is necessary with CD. Several enzyme or lactase supplements are available over-the-counter without a prescription, including Lactaid and Lactaid Ultra. These lactase-containing pills are taken at the time of eating a dairy product. Alternatively, drops of liquid enzyme can be added to milk to help predigest the offending lactose. Also, most supermarkets sell reduced-lactose or lactose-free milk. Be careful, though: Lactose intolerance exists along a spectrum. Some people have mild lactose sensitivity and need to consume a large amount of dairy-containing products to develop symptoms; others are very sensitive and get sick even when they consume only tiny amounts of lactose. Lactaid milk has reduced lactose but is not completely free of this sugar, so it will cause symptoms in individuals who are extremely lactose intolerant. Other options include soy-based milk, which does not contain any lactose.

17. Should all people with lactose intolerance be checked for celiac disease?

This is a tough question, and there is no "textbook" answer. The short answer is probably no, albeit with an explanation and a disclaimer. As mentioned in Question 16, lactose intolerance is very common. I tell my patients to simply avoid milk and dairy products or to take the enzyme supplements. If this approach works adequately, no further evaluation is needed. If patients continue to have bloating, gas, and diarrhea despite a lactose-restricted diet, then they should be checked for CD. If there is a family history of CD and a family member is lactose intolerant, then patients should have the blood test for CD.

Weight loss for any patient is a "red flag": People with lactose intolerance should not have unexplained weight loss. In such a case, they should seek medical attention and be checked for CD. Because CD is common among persons of Irish, Italian, and French Canadian heritage, the presence of lactose intolerance also warrants a check for CD in such individuals. If an unexplained anemia is present in the setting of lactose intolerance, then CD should be ruled out.

18. What is the association between anemia and celiac disease?

Anemia or a low blood count goes hand-in-hand with CD and is the most common blood abnormality and clue. Doctors routinely perform a **complete blood count (CBC)** when screening their patients; indeed, this test is usually part of the blood work that is ordered during an annual physical. The CBC consists of several items:

- A white blood cell (WBC) count, which counts the blood cells that fight infection
- A platelet (PLT) count, which counts the cells that help the blood clot
- A red blood cell (RBC) count

Complete blood count (CBC)

A type of blood test that gives information on anemia, infection, and the body's ability to stop bleeding. Measurements of hemoglobin (Hg) and hematocrit (HCT) are part of a CBC.

Red blood cells contain hemoglobin, an iron-containing protein that carries oxygen from the lungs to the rest of the body. The CBC gives several measurements pertaining to the red blood cells—namely, the hemoglobin level (Hb), the hematocrit level (HCT), and a description of how the red blood cells look. Normally, red blood cells are round (like a dinner plate); in CD, however, they may be abnormally small or large or have a bizarre appearance.

If any of these RBC tests are abnormal, then an anemia is diagnosed. Anemia simply means a low or abnormal amount of red blood cells. General symptoms of anemia include fatigue, tiredness, and shortness of breath. Many causes of anemia

Symptoms and Manifestations

are possible, which can be grouped into three categories: abnormal production of red blood cells, loss of red blood cells (bleeding), or shortened red blood cell lifespan.

Red blood cell production in the bone marrow is very complicated, and a number of "ingredients" are required to carry out this process correctly. In particular, an adequate supply of iron is needed to make hemoglobin. Iron is acquired in the diet from meats and green leafy vegetables such as spinach. It is processed in the stomach and first part of the small intestine where iron is released or made usable. Iron absorption from the gut occurs in the first parts of the small intestine, called the **duodenum** and the proximal **jejunum**. This is the part of the gut that is most commonly damaged by CD, resulting in decreased or inadequate iron absorption and anemia. For this reason, the medical evaluation of an unexplained iron-deficiency anemia includes checking for CD. Studies of asymptomatic patients with iron-deficiency anemia have found rates of CD ranging from 2.8 percent to 8.7 percent.

Duodenum

The first part of the small intestine.

Jejunum

The middle part of the small intestine.

Iron-deficiency anemia can be caused by chronic blood losses consisting of small-quantity but long-duration bleeding. The end result is the loss of bodily iron stores and anemia. A classic example occurs in colon cancer, where microscopic, slow bleeding can be ongoing for months to years. Part of the evaluation for iron-deficiency anemia is a colonoscopy to check for cancer and an upper GI endoscopy to check for ulcers and take a small intestine biopsy for CD. Chronic bleeding can be present in CD because of the disease-related inflammation and damage to the gut lining, which allows for microscopic bleeding.

The diet must include adequate amounts of vitamin B_{12} to ensure normal red blood cell production. Sources of vitamin B_{12} include meats and legume vegetables. Absorption of this vitamin by the gut is complicated and requires several coordinated steps. Because vitamin B_{12} processing is so complicated and a defect at any step along the way results in a deficiency,

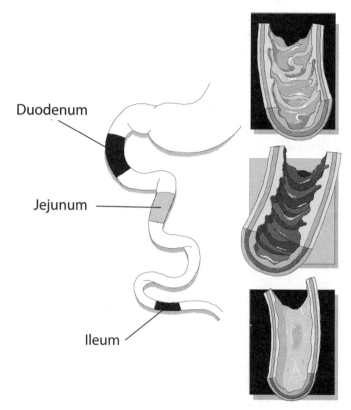

Duodenum

Jejunum

Ileum

Figure 3   Cartoon of the parts of the small intestine, the duodenum, jejunum, and ileum.

faulty processing is a frequent abnormality in CD. Vitamin B_{12} is absorbed from a part of the small intestine called the **ileum.** Although most nutrients can be absorbed anywhere in the small intestine, there are exceptions—namely, iron and vitamin B_{12}. In my practice, I recommend that all CD patients have their vitamin B_{12} levels checked annually. If levels are low, patients are started on monthly B_{12} shots, although B_{12} absorption should improve with a gluten-free diet. Eventually, it may be possible to switch to an oral supplement if blood levels are followed and remain stable. A vitamin B_{12} deficiency can result in anemia, numbness or tingling of the hands and feet, difficulty walking (including falls), and neurologic damage that, if caught early, can be treated.

Ileum

The last part of the small intestine, found just before the colon.

Folic acid (also known as **folate**) is another vitamin whose level is affected by CD. This nutrient, which is needed for red blood cell production, is both available from the diet and produced by intestinal bacteria; hence a folic acid deficiency is less common than an iron or vitamin B_{12} deficiency. Supplements are easily taken by mouth if needed, and levels should be checked upon the initial diagnosis of CD and then annually thereafter.

The spleen is an organ in the abdomen that serves to filter the blood and remove old or damaged red blood cells; in this way, it helps protect the body against infection. The spleen can be damaged in CD, which may potentially shorten the lifespan of red blood cells and thereby contribute to anemia.

19. What is the association between fertility and celiac disease?

Fertility is the ability for a woman to become pregnant, to maintain the pregnancy, and to ultimately have a child. Both female and male factors affect this process, and many issues aside from CD may impair fertility. Women with undiagnosed or untreated CD, however, often have irregularities related to their menstrual periods. For example, CD can cause a delay (on average, lasting one year) in adolescent girls having their first period. **Amenorrhea** (lack of a menstrual period for three months or more) is also more common in women with untreated CD. Menopause may also occur several years earlier than normal in women with untreated CD. All of these factors contribute to decreasing the "reproductive lifespan" of a woman with untreated CD.

Women with untreated CD may also have an impaired ability to become pregnant and to carry the pregnancy to term. Spontaneous pregnancy loss—particularly within the first trimester—is twice as common in those patients with CD on a gluten-containing diet versus those patients with CD on a gluten-free diet. Repeated unexplained miscarriages may be a sign of CD, so testing should be part of the evaluation for infertility. Babies born to women with untreated CD are at increased risk of **intrauterine growth retardation** and hence are often small compared to the "normal" expected size and weight.

Men can also experience sexual impairment related to CD. Puberty and the development of secondary sex characteristics can be delayed in CD. Untreated CD can result in lower sperm counts and abnormal sperm, both of which decrease fertility. Treatment of CD with a gluten-free diet will improve both female and male fertility and normalize these problems.

20. What is the association between psychiatric/neurologic disease and celiac disease?

Celiac disease is a systemic illness, meaning it involves the whole body and can affect many different organ systems. It can affect both the central and peripheral nervous systems, resulting in psychiatric and neurologic disease. Several well-defined neurologic manifestations of CD are distinguished. **Ataxia** is difficulty walking or standing with impaired balance. **Peripheral neuropathies** include numbness and tingling of the hands and/or feet. Headaches or migraines, paralysis, dementia, and seizures have well-recognized associations with CD. Abnormalities seen on CAT scans of these patients' brains may include calcium deposits and atrophy.

A recent study of 312 neurology patients with gluten allergy revealed that 47 percent had gluten-induced ataxia, 37 percent had peripheral neuropathy, 10 percent had **encephalopathy** (confusion), and 5 percent had **myopathy** (muscle inflammation and weakness). In this study, treatment with a gluten-free diet stabilized or improved patients' symptoms within one year; the sooner the diet was started, the better patients did.

Intrauterine growth retardation
Delayed fetal growth.

Ataxia
Difficulty walking, characterized by a staggering gait.

Peripheral neuropathy
Numbness or tingling in the arms and legs.

Encephalopathy
Mental confusion

Myopathy
An inflammatory condition affecting the muscles.

Symptoms and Manifestations

Magnetic resonance imaging (MRI) demonstrated atrophy of the cerebellum (the part of the brain responsible for coordinated movement) in 60 percent of the patients. Most of the patients tested positive for antigliadin antibodies and did not have any GI symptoms.

The cause of celiac-associated neurologic disease is probably multifactorial. Vitamin deficiencies are most likely, given that vitamin B$_{12}$ deficiency causes ataxia and peripheral neuropathy. **Thiamine** deficiency can cause **dry beri beri,** which is characterized by difficulty with memory, difficulty walking, and confusion. Low levels of calcium, magnesium, phosphorus, and potassium may lead to muscle weakness, cramps, and dysfunction. Activation of the immune system with antibody production and increased inflammation may also play a role in the development of neurologic disease. Celiac disease is an autoimmune disease, as are several neurologic disorders that are linked to gluten sensitivity and positive antibodies.

Chronic illness, pain, fatigue, itchy rash, and diarrhea are very common causes of depression in patients with CD. Given the usual 8- to 10-year delay in diagnosis of CD, the association between the two diseases is quite strong. Depression may follow the initial diagnosis: Learning you have a chronic disease and will require a lifelong gluten-free diet can be staggering. Vitamin deficiencies, weakness and fatigue from malnutrition, and associated medical conditions such as an underactive thyroid may also contribute to depression. Depression is the most common psychiatric manifestation of CD.

21. What is the association between bone disease/osteoporosis and celiac disease?

Osteoporosis is a thinning of the bones that can result in a tendency toward bone fractures and/or a loss of height owing to spontaneous spine fractures. Fractures may range from minimal trauma from stubbing your toe to a hip fracture from a minor fall that requires surgery. Risk factors for osteoporosis

Thiamine

An essential vitamin that can be deficient in celiac disease.

Dry beri beri

A vitamin deficiency of thiamine characterized by neurologic symptoms.

Fat-soluble vitamin

A vitamin that is absorbed with fat. Fat-soluble vitamins include vitamins A, D, E, and K.

include female sex, Caucasian ethnicity, thin build, smoking, low-calcium or low-vitamin D diet (such as a dairy-restricted diet in a lactose-intolerant person), family history of osteoporosis, living in a low-sun-exposure climate, and diseases of the small intestine such as CD. Frequently, patients with osteoporosis are screened for, and found to have, CD. These people are generally asymptomatic and have no gastrointestinal symptoms. Rates of CD in studies of these patients vary from 1 percent to 3.4 percent.

Vitamin D and calcium are both derived from the diet, and both are needed to maintain bone strength and health. In CD, normal digestion and absorption of dietary fat are reduced, manifesting as abnormal stools and diarrhea. Vitamin D is a **fat-soluble vitamin,** meaning it is taken up with fats; thus its absorption is reduced in CD as well. Similarly, absorption of dietary calcium is linked to fat, and it affects bone health in multiple ways. Bone is the main reservoir for calcium in the body, and blood calcium levels are normally tightly controlled. Signs of a low blood calcium level include an uncontrollable muscle twitching called **tetany.** When dietary absorption calcium is inadequate and levels drop, then calcium is released from bone. If this process continues for a prolonged period of time, ultimately the bone will thin. Bone thinning in children is called **rickets** but is rare in our era of vitamin D–supplemented foods (for example, dairy products typically contain extra vitamin D). Mild thinning of the bones in adults is called **osteopenia;** more significant thinning with increased fractures is termed osteoporosis. The chronic leaching of calcium from bone is called secondary **hyperparathyroidism.**

All patients diagnosed with CD should have an evaluation for bone health called a **bone density scan** or **DEXA scan.** This kind of testing is helpful to determine whether bone disease has developed and can be done every year or two to monitor the effectiveness of the patient's treatment for osteoporosis. Early treatments include taking calcium and vitamin D supplements, quitting smoking, engaging in exercise,

Symptoms and Manifestations

Tetany

A spasm of the muscles caused by very low blood calcium levels.

Rickets

A vitamin D deficiency found in children with malformed bones.

Osteopenia

Mild thinning of the bones. It is treated with calcium and vitamin D supplements.

Hyperpara-thyroidism

A condition caused by low vitamin D levels that predisposes a person to osteoporosis.

Bone density scan

An x-ray test used to measure the mineral content of bone and diagnose osteoporosis and the risk of fracture.

DEXA scan

A test that measures bone mineral content, risk of fracture, and osteoporosis.

avoiding drugs that cause osteoporosis (such as steroids), and treating any underlying intestinal disorders. If osteoporosis has developed, then medications called bisphosphonates may be administered; examples include Fosamax, Boniva, and Zometa. Your doctor may prescribe these medications or refer you to a physician who specializes in bone health, such as an **endocrinologist** or **rheumatologist**.

In my practice, when I make a new diagnosis of CD, I order blood work that includes a vitamin D level and a calcium level; patients also undergo a bone density test (a DEXA scan). All patients are asked to take supplements consisting of 1200 to 1600 mg of calcium and 800 IU of vitamin D per day. These supplements are available over the counter, and some combinations include both calcium and vitamin D in a single pill. Gluten-free examples are Caltrate, Citracal, and Viactiv. If the patient's vitamin D levels are very low, then prescription vitamin D may be required. Testing should be repeated every one to two years to follow the results of treatment, with tests including both the bone density test and blood tests for both calcium and vitamin D.

Children or adolescents with CD may improve their bone density by adhering to a gluten-free diet. They may not require any further treatment other than some calcium and vitamin D supplements.

Marye comments:

My bone density test results were okay, but high dosages of vitamin D were prescribed for me.

22. Is there an association between liver abnormalities and celiac disease?

The **liver** is an organ in the abdomen that assists in processing food, eliminating toxins from the body, and maintaining the immune system's ability to fight infection. Many different diseases affect the liver. Generally, they cause inflammation of

Endocrinologist

A doctor who specializes in the treatment of glandular disorders such as diabetes, thyroid disease, and osteoporosis.

Rheumatologist

A doctor who specializes in the treatment of muscle, bone, and joint diseases.

Liver

An organ in the abdomen that processes nutrients, makes bile, has immune function, and makes proteins.

Hepatitis

An inflammatory condition of the liver that can be chronic, resulting in scarring (cirrhosis) and jaundice.

Jaundice

The symptoms of turning yellow and having dark, tea-colored urine that occur in conjunction with liver disease or hepatitis.

the liver, a condition called **hepatitis.** Typical causes of hepatitis are viral infections of the liver such as with the hepatitis A, B, or C virus. All of these problems lead to increased liver tests, possible **jaundice** (turning yellow), nausea, vomiting, malaise, and occasionally some discomfort in the upper-right side of the abdomen. Other causes of hepatitis are not related to infections, such as reactions to medications, herbs or nutritional supplements, and alcohol.

In an autoimmune disease, the body identifies part of itself as foreign and attacks the supposed "invader"; this reaction can also cause hepatitis. As mentioned previously, CD is an autoimmune disease. Examples of **autoimmune liver diseases** include **autoimmune hepatitis (AIH), primary biliary cirrhosis,** and **primary sclerosing cholangitis,** to name a few. These diseases may have few or no symptoms or may result in slow, progressive damage to the liver with the development of **cirrhosis.** In cirrhosis, the liver becomes scarred and cannot perform its usual function; this disease increases a person's risk of getting cancer of the liver. Autoimmune diseases tend to occur together. Consequently, if you have one autoimmune disease such as CD, you may have an increased risk of developing another one. Autoimmune liver disease is usually treatable with medication. A gluten-free diet is not helpful.

Another liver disorder that generally has no symptoms is **fatty liver disease.** As mentioned earlier, two thirds of Americans are overweight and one third are obese (that is, roughly 30 pounds overweight). When a person is overweight, fat may be deposited in the liver. This fat may produce inflammation with abnormal blood liver tests, hepatitis, and (rarely) development of cirrhosis. Less commonly, rapid weight loss and being underweight may cause fatty liver disease, possibly related to abnormal liver processing of nutrients from the diet. This phenomenon occurs in CD, so frequently patients who are newly diagnosed with CD have abnormal liver tests. Thankfully this condition usually goes away with stabilization of weight loss upon switching to a gluten-free diet.

Autoimmune liver disease

See *Autoimmune hepatitis.*

Autoimmune hepatitis (AIH)

A chronic, progressive inflammatory disease of the liver in which the body attacks itself. It can result in cirrhosis.

Primary biliary cirrhosis

A chronic inflammatory condition of the liver that tends to occur in women and may be associated with celiac disease.

Primary sclerosing cholangitis

A chronic inflammatory condition of the liver characterized by scarring of the bile ducts.

Cirrhosis

An advanced form of liver disease characterized by scarring of the liver and an increased risk of liver failure, cancer, and death.

Fatty liver disease

An inflammatory disease of the liver caused by excessive deposits of fat in the liver.

Because of the association of CD with autoimmune disease and fatty liver disease, in my practice I always check a set of liver tests in a patient with newly diagnosed CD. The liver tests actually comprise a panel of several blood tests and can give the doctor a lot of information. Some tests can indicate whether inflammation of the liver is present; others provide information on the patient's nutritional status. Both issues are important in CD, as abnormalities can give clues about the presence of other diseases.

The second issue regarding liver tests and CD is sort of the opposite of the above. Liver test abnormalities sometimes have a reason like excessive alcohol use or hepatitis. Nevertheless, the cause of these abnormalities is often unknown. Because CD is so common, I recommend checking patients with abnormal liver tests for CD. This is another way to identify patients with otherwise asymptomatic CD.

Marye comments:

I did have my liver functions tested frequently prior to being diagnosed with celiac disease.

23. What is the association between cancer and celiac disease?

Mortality
Death rate.

Non-Hodgkin's lymphoma (NHL)
A type of lymphoma.

Lymphoma
A cancer generally affecting the lymph nodes that can involve any part of the body.

Several medical studies have found that people with CD have a higher **mortality** (death rate) compared to individuals without CD. This excess death rate was related to two issues: severe malabsorption and increased cancer rate. In particular, the presence of the cancer called **non-Hodgkin's lymphoma (NHL)** increased the death rate by about 2.5 times.

Lymphoma comprises several types of cancer of the lymph nodes; it can involve a single lymph node, multiple lymph nodes, or any organ, including the gut. There tends to be an increase in the rate at which patients are diagnosed with lymphoma around the same time that they are diagnosed with

CD. This linkage may be because the patient is seeing a doctor and undergoing a medical evaluation and testing that uncovers the cancer or because the cancer initiated the CD.

Non-Hodgkin's lymphoma is a group of several different cancers that are increased in the setting of CD. One type of NHL called **enteropathy-associated T-cell lymphoma (EATL)** involves the small intestine; it is fairly specific to CD but is rare. Studies suggest that the risk of lymphoma is 2.5 to 6.5 times greater in patients with CD, but that fewer than half of these lymphomas involve EATL. Most lymphomas are treatable, which explains why the risk of lymphoma and the death rate from CD are different: Most patients do not die from their lymphoma. By contrast, EATL is very difficult to treat and often proves fatal.

Enteropathy-associated T-cell lymphoma (EATL)

A type of T-cell lymphoma of the small intestine that can, on rare occasions, be a complication of celiac disease.

The relationship between cancer and CD comes up frequently in the physician's office as patients ask about complications of CD. They may also search the Internet, see data about the increased risk of cancer in conjunction with CD, and become concerned. First, all of these cancers are relatively rare. In my more than 10 years of personal experience in my group of about 20 **gastroenterologists** caring for hundreds of patients with CD, we have seen only one case of EATL. Second, following a strict gluten-free diet has been shown to decrease a person's risk of developing NHL and EATL. One study found that the same cancer rate in patients with CD who followed a strict gluten-free diet as in people without CD. This is one of the main reasons I recommend that all patients with CD go on a gluten-free diet (and minimize cheating).

Gastroenterologist

A doctor who specializes in treating diseases of the intestine, stomach, esophagus, liver, and pancreas and who does endoscopic procedures related to these organs.

24. Which diarrheal diseases can occur in conjunction with celiac disease?

There are many causes of diarrhea in patients with CD. Obviously, the CD itself may cause the diarrhea when fluid leaks from the small intestine or when food or fat is poorly absorbed. Known or unknown gluten ingestion can fuel this process, with repeated, ongoing damage to the small intestine resulting in chronic diarrhea. In addition, complications of CD such as refractory sprue, collagenous sprue, and EATL may not respond to a gluten-free diet and may produce diarrhea associated with weight loss.

As discussed in Question 16, lactose intolerance is a common cause of diarrhea in patients with new CD. In this condition, the person suffers a temporary or permanent loss of the gut enzyme that aids in digesting lactose (a sugar found in milk). The small intestine does not process dietary lactose from dairy products in such cases, so the sugar reaches the colon. There, it is used by colonic bacteria, which results in gas, cramps, and diarrhea. Lactose intolerance is treated either by avoiding dairy products or by taking enzyme supplements to help digest the lactose.

Irritable bowel syndrome (IBS; see Question 15) is the most common cause of diarrhea. We do not really know why IBS causes diarrhea, but the likely culprit is abnormal intestinal motility or pumping. This problem may be caused by consumption of foods that may stimulate the gut—for example, fatty foods, caffeine, chocolate, spicy foods, and alcohol. Avoiding these foods is the first choice for treatment. If this measure fails, then antidiarrheal medications such as over-the-counter kaopectate and Imodium or prescription lomotil can help.

Normally, bacteria live in the **large intestine** or **colon,** where they help digest food and produce some key vitamins. Several barriers keep the bacteria in the colon, thereby preventing them from moving into the small intestine. Celiac disease damages the small intestine lining and also affects the normal motility of the gut, which moves things downstream from your mouth to bottom. In CD, these barriers can break down, allowing bacteria to populate the small intestine. This phenomenon is called **small intestine bacterial overgrowth (SIBO)** or just bacterial overgrowth. Symptoms of SIBO

Large intestine
The colon.

Colon
The large intestine, which functions to process and store wastes.

Small intestinal bacterial overgrowth (SIBO)
Overgrowth of the number and type of bacteria in the small intestine, causing diarrhea, weight loss, and vitamin deficiencies.

include diarrhea, gas, weight loss, and anemia. This problem frequently occurs commonly in new CD and may explain ongoing symptoms despite consumption of a gluten-free diet. Your doctor should test you for SIBO and, if found, can treat it with antibiotics.

Digestion and processing of food for absorption is a very complicated process that requires the coordinated activity of several organs. **Bile** is a liquid that is produced in the liver, stored in the gallbladder, and released after a meal into the gut. The bile mixes with food and helps make dietary fat available for absorption. The bile is then itself absorbed and reused. In CD, the site for bile absorption can be damaged, so that bile passes into the colon. The result is burning, watery diarrhea (**bile salt diarrhea**). This condition is easily treatable by your doctor.

The **thyroid** is a gland in the neck that makes hormones that regulate body functions almost like the thermostat in your house. Most thyroid diseases are autoimmune in nature—the body attacks itself. Likewise, CD is an autoimmune disease and very commonly is associated with thyroid problems. Autoimmune thyroid disease can result from either an overactive or an underactive thyroid and can occur years before or after the diagnosis of CD. Symptoms of an overactive thyroid include weight loss, palpitations, anxiety, intolerance to hot weather, and diarrhea. This condition is easily evaluated with a blood test and is treatable with medicine.

Frequently, patients are referred to a gastroenterologist for chronic diarrhea. Part of this evaluation may be a colonoscopy —a test that examines the lining of the large intestine with an endoscope and allows for taking biopsies (tissue samples). If the colonoscopy looks normal but the biopsy reveals inflammation, the person has microscopic colitis. Microscopic colitis is common in CD and manifests as diarrhea. All patients with microscopic colitis should be checked for CD. Conversely, individuals with CD who are following a gluten-free diet

Bile
A green liquid made by the liver and stored in the gallbladder that helps to digest fats.

Bile salt diarrhea
A chronic diarrheal illness caused by poor absorption of bile. It is typically treated with cholestyramine.

Thyroid
A gland in the neck that is the body's thermostat and controls metabolism.

Symptoms and Manifestations

yet have diarrhea should have a colonoscopy to check for microscopic colitis. Patients with microscopic colitis generally do not lose weight, so any weight loss should also prompt an evaluation for something else like CD. In my practice, I have seen several patients who were treated by GI doctors for years with intractable symptoms of diarrhea, weight loss, vitamin deficiencies, and muscle weakness and who have been diagnosed with microscopic colitis, only to discover that they actually have CD. Once the correct diagnosis is made, a gluten-free diet often resolves the GI symptoms.

25. Can I have a sensitivity to gluten but not have celiac disease?

The short answer is yes, but this is a complicated issue. Gluten is a difficult protein to digest, and trouble with its processing frequently can produce symptoms even in the absence of CD. Patients with IBS may react to gluten and, as mentioned in Question 15, may benefit from avoiding gluten-containing products such as pasta.

Celiac disease, however, is an allergy manifested by inflammation and changes in the small intestine after consuming gluten-containing food. An allergy arises when the body responds to an offending agent by activating the immune system. Examples of this abnormal immune response include swelling, rash, and difficulty breathing after a bee sting or getting an itchy rash after taking a medication to which you are allergic.

Sensitivity, by contrast, is a reaction to something that does not involve the immune system. Examples include consuming too much caffeinated coffee, which may cause diarrhea, or eating a large fatty meal, which may produce cramps and diarrhea. These activities stimulate the gut directly and do not cause inflammation. Gluten can have a similar effect because it is very dense and **osmotically active**—it pulls water into the gut to dilute it, resulting in cramps and diarrhea. Patients

Osmotically active

The condition in which a substance draws water into the gut.

with gluten sensitivity do not need to follow an absolute gluten-free diet but rather may improve with gluten reduction or restriction.

The confusion regarding the answer to this question arises because sometimes CD can be very challenging to diagnose and may seem confusing to patients, doctors, and alternative or holistic practitioners alike. Despite the fact that both are treated with a gluten restriction, gluten sensitivity and CD are different conditions.

Several blood tests can be used to diagnose CD, though some are more helpful than others. Some are nonspecific; if positive, they may or may not indicate CD. Such a result may prompt the patient to receive a false diagnosis of CD when it is not really present. (These blood tests are discussed further in Part 4.) For this reason, I never recommend a trial of a gluten-free diet as a way to determine whether a patient has CD. If he or she responds to this diet, a person who actually has IBS may be mistakenly labeled as having CD and placed on an unnecessary lifelong gluten-free diet, when avoidance of pasta or breads may be sufficient. Gluten-sensitive patients without CD do not develop any of the associated complications of CD such as anemia, osteoporosis, weight loss, and infertility.

26. Which other diseases can mimic celiac disease?

Celiac disease has many manifestations, spanning from no symptoms to life-threatening disease. Because of the variability in symptoms, which inspires CD's label of "the great masquerader," it takes on average eight years to make the correct diagnosis. Indeed, CD is frequently mistaken or misdiagnosed as another disease process. For individuals with typical GI symptoms of bloating, cramps, and diarrhea, for example, CD is commonly misdiagnosed as IBS. Gluten sensitivity, which usually features the same constellation of symptoms, can also be confused with CD.

Many diseases of the small intestine can be confused with CD, especially when the patient experiences weight loss. For example, **Crohn's disease,** an inflammatory disorder that can involve any part of the gut, including the small intestine, commonly causes diarrhea, bloating, weight loss, and anemia. The diagnosis of Crohn's disease is usually made by barium x-rays of the small or large intestine or by colonoscopy. These studies will show ulcers and nodularity of the affected gut, along with possible **strictures** (narrowing of the intestine). Biopsies show inflammation of the lining of the gut, which is different from the inflammation seen in CD.

Diseases that complicate CD can add confusion to the picture. Microscopic colitis, for example, causes chronic watery diarrhea and can affect patients with or without CD. Small intestine bacterial overgrowth with diarrhea, bloating, weight loss, and anemia also may or may not occur with CD. Because of these disease associations, blood testing for CD must be performed to clarify the diagnosis.

Several infectious diseases involving the small intestine can mimic CD. Tropical sprue is an infectious disease that is usually acquired after a trip to the tropics. Its symptoms are the same as those seen with CD, and the small intestine biopsies for both diseases look similar; nevertheless, the treatments for tropical sprue and non-tropical sprue (CD) are quite different despite their similar names. In case of tropical sprue, the patient's history generally includes a trip to the Caribbean or the Far East, and blood tests for CD are negative. Tropical sprue usually improves with antibiotics and does not require following a gluten-free diet. And despite the similar names, the diseases are completely different.

Whipple's disease is another infectious disease that involves the small intestine and causes weight loss and diarrhea. Its diagnosis is confirmed by biopsy of the small intestine, as the bacteria can be visualized under the microscope. Whipple's disease is treated with antibiotics.

Crohn's disease

An autoimmune inflammatory disease that can affect any part of the gastrointestinal tract. Crohn's disease of the small intestine can mimic celiac disease.

Stricture

A narrowing of the intestine.

Whipple's disease

An infectious disease of the small intestine characterized by gastrointestinal and neurologic symptoms.

Tuberculosis is an infection that usually involves the lungs. It results in a chronic cough and weight loss, but rarely patients can have intestinal involvement with CD-type symptoms. Imaging, colonoscopy, biopsy, and cultures help to differentiate the two diseases. Treatment for tuberculosis consists of a prolonged course of antibiotics.

Several different parasites can infect the small intestine and produce symptoms similar to those seen with CD. *Giardia* is a parasite that is usually acquired by drinking contaminated or unprocessed water. A typical history is drinking lake or stream water from northern New England or contaminated water from some of the former Soviet republics. Infections can be chronic, lasting years to decades, and produce bloating, gas, diarrhea, and sometimes weight loss. Diagnosis is made by examining the patient's stool under the microscope or by sampling fluid or tissue from the small intestine and examining it for *Giardia*. A blood test is also available for diagnosis of this infection.

Human immunodeficiency virus (HIV), the infectious organism that causes acquired immunodeficiency syndrome (AIDS), commonly causes diarrhea and weight loss, among its many other symptoms. Testing for HIV should be considered especially if the patient has known risk factors such as prior blood transfusion, history of intravenous drug use with needle sharing, unprotected sex, or multiple sexual partners. HIV can predispose the affected individual to parasitic infections or lymphoma of the small intestine; stool examination and biopsies can help to diagnose its presence.

Hyperthyroidism (an overactive thyroid) causes diarrhea and weight loss, thereby mimicking CD. Medical evaluation of chronic diarrhea includes blood testing for thyroid problems. As mentioned in Question 24, thyroid disease is commonly associated with CD. For this reason, when seeing a new patient with chronic diarrhea, I always perform blood testing for both thyroid disease and CD.

Tuberculosis
A chronic infectious disease that requires prolonged antibiotics for treatment.

Giardia
A parasite that is usually acquired from contaminated water and that infects the intestine, where it causes symptoms similar to those seen with celiac disease (diarrhea, weight loss, and bloating).

Human immunodeficiency virus (HIV)
The causative virus in AIDS.

Hyperthyroidism
A condition in which an overactive thyroid causes diarrhea, weight loss, palpitations, and intolerance to heat. Also known as Graves' disease.

Symptoms and Manifestations

The gut requires many components for normal digestion. In particular, bile helps break down large particles of fat into a more digestible form. Bile is produced in the liver and stored in the gallbladder. After a meal, the gallbladder contracts, moving the bile into the duodenum to mix with food. More than 90 percent of the bile in the intestine is absorbed and reused. However, if the bile is not normally absorbed in the small intestine, it can reach the colon or large intestine. Bile is very irritating to the colon and can cause burning, watery diarrhea called bile salt diarrhea. Bile salt diarrhea can occur either spontaneously or after the gallbladder is removed. In addition, CD can cause bile salt diarrhea.

Because CD has many extra-intestinal (non-gut) manifestations, the picture it presents can really get confusing. Its association with psychiatric illness, fertility, skin diseases, anemia, thyroid disease, bone disease, and liver disease all warrant careful evaluation by a doctor. Given that diagnosis of CD is easy with blood testing, this possibility should be considered in any of these conditions, and you might request testing if you have one of them.

PART THREE

Children and Celiac Disease

Do children get celiac disease?

Which diseases are associated with celiac disease in children?

What are the complications of celiac disease in children?

More . . .

27. Do children get celiac disease?

Celiac disease is well recognized in children, and can occur in those as young as several months old. In 1888, Samuel Gee gave a lecture at the Hospital for Sick Children in London, titled the "Coeliac Affection," in which he described the disease:

There is a kind of chronic indigestion in persons of all ages, yet is especially apt to affect children between one and five years old. Faeces (bowel movements) being loose, not formed, more bulky than the food would seem to account for. Errors in the diet may perhaps be a cause, but what error?

Rice

A gluten-free grain.

Sago

A gluten-free grain.

Gee went further by stating that highly starched foods—for example, **rice, sago,** and corn-flour—were "unfit" for consumption. He did not make the link between gluten and sprue but did understand that some component of the diet was toxic for these children.

It was not until the 1940s, during World War II, that the cause of CD was found to be gluten. Dr. Willem Dicke, a Dutch pediatrician, found that during food shortages (namely, shortages of breads and cereals), children with relapsing diarrhea improved. After the war, when wheat products became more widely available, Dicke did studies on sick children by varying their diet and measuring the amount of stool produced. He found that wheat, rye, barley, and, to a lesser degree, oats triggered malabsorption and that the patients' symptoms improved with these foods removed from the diet. A few years later it was discovered that gluten—a protein in these grains—was the toxic agent.

Although many studies have looked at the rate of CD in population-based screenings, most of these investigations involved adults. The largest pediatric study was done on 17,200 Italian school children, ranging from age 6 to 15. The rate of CD was found to be 1 in 184 children, and most children who tested positive for the disease had few or no symptoms. This result is somewhat concerning, as most of the children were asymptomatic and likely would never have been diagnosed with any problems. This raises the question of whether there are different "kinds" of CD based on the presence or absence of symptoms. The Italian study found that the ratio of asymptomatic to symptomatic children was 7:1. This relationship is analogous to an iceberg: Only a small number of symptomatic cases are visible, with most cases floating out of sight under the water line.

Marye comments:

One of the celiac support groups that I attend includes many parents. Their children have the disease, but the parents do not, nor are they aware of anyone else in their family who has the disease. Today, the food choices are easier for children with celiac disease, because many gluten-free breads, cereals, cookies, and cold cuts are available.

28. What are the manifestations of celiac disease in children?

There are four major types of CD in children:

- Classical CD with gastrointestinal symptoms usually appears at 6 months to 2 years and is characterized by diarrhea, poor growth and weight gain, bloating, and irritability.
- **Nonclassical CD** tends to affect older children (5 to 7 years). Its symptoms may include abdominal symptoms, tooth abnormalities, short stature, delayed puberty, and rashes.
- Silent CD is asymptomatic, yet affected children have positive blood tests for CD and abnormal small intestinal biopsies. These children are usually found by screening those deemed to be at high risk for the disease—for example, the child of a parent with known CD.

Nonclassical celiac disease

Celiac disease with atypical or no manifestations.

Children and Celiac Disease

- Latent or potential CD is found in children who have positive blood tests for CD and the appropriate genetic predisposition (that is, the HLA-DQ2 or HLA-DQ8 gene). Intestinal biopsies in potential CD patients are normal or minimally abnormal.

The Italian children's celiac study found that only 17 percent of children tested were symptomatic; 83 percent had no symptoms. These 83 percent of children are below the water line of the iceberg (Figure 4). The general recommendation is that children with latent or potential CD should not go on a gluten-free diet because the benefit of doing so is unknown. Symptomatic disease is split between those with classic and nonclassic manifestations. Many of the pediatric symptoms are similar to those in adults, but some are unique to children. Given that a large percentage of children are asymptomatic, the spectrum pediatric disease is even wider than that of adults, making diagnosis in the younger age group even more difficult.

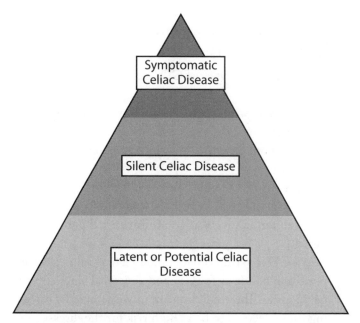

Figure 4 **The celiac iceberg. The visible part of the iceberg is the darkest gray area, indicating symptomatic celiac disease.**

Table 8   Manifestations of Celiac Disease in Children

Classic Symptoms
Chronic diarrhea
Failure to thrive
Irritability
Weight loss
Poor feeding
Abdominal bloating
Abdominal pain

Nonclassic Symptoms
Anemia
Impaired growth with short stature
Mouth ulcers
Dental abnormalities
Delayed puberty
Dermatitis herpetiformis
Depression
Rickets (vitamin D deficiency)
Seizures
Liver abnormalities

29. Which diseases are associated with celiac disease in children?

Many diseases are associated with CD in children. In general, they can be broken out into two groups: diseases that are genetically associated with CD and autoimmune-mediated diseases.

Genetic Diseases

There is a strong association of CD with **Down syndrome,** a link that has been well studied. Down syndrome (also called **trisomy 21**) is a genetic abnormality that is acquired early in fetal development shortly after the woman's egg is fertilized. An affected child carries an extra copy of the twenty-first gene. This mutation results in mental retardation, developmental delay, and an abnormal-appearing face. Various studies on children with Down syndrome have demonstrated that the rate of CD in this population ranges between 3.2 percent and 10.3 percent—is 100-fold higher risk than for the general population. Children with the combination of Down syndrome and CD may exhibit variable symptoms, which may

Down syndrome

A syndrome of mental retardation that is present at birth. There is a very strong association between Down syndrome and celiac disease. Also called trisomy 21.

Children and Celiac Disease

55

be attributed to the Down syndrome, or they might have no GI symptoms. Testing and establishing a diagnosis of CD and implementing a gluten-free diet can improve the quality of life for these children. Screening children with Down syndrome for CD with blood testing should be considered and discussed with your pediatrician.

Williams syndrome

A rare genetic disorder of mental retardation that is highly associated with celiac disease.

Williams syndrome is a rare genetic syndrome that is characterized by a variable degree of mental retardation, learning difficulties, a distinct facial appearance, and a unique personality trait of over-friendliness. More than half of all children with this syndrome have attention-deficit disorder. Studies demonstrate that as many as 10 percent of children with Williams syndrome will test positive for CD. Blood antibody testing for CD should be considered for these children.

Turner syndrome

A syndrome present at birth that affects females and is highly associated with celiac disease.

Turner syndrome is a rare genetic disorder that affects only females. It is characterized by growth retardation, a webbed (wide) neck, and lack of ovarian development. Studies of children with Turner syndrome showed a 10.6 percent rate of CD. A frequent manifestation of this syndrome is growth retardation, which can be treated with growth hormone shots to stimulate growth. Some authors recommend testing for CD in children with Turner syndrome who demonstrate growth retardation prior to the initiation of growth hormone therapy because those with CD may respond to the gluten-free diet, thereby improving growth.

Selective IgA deficiency is a defect of the immune system dating from birth that results in increased risk of recurrent ear, sinus, and lung infections. Some people with selective IgA deficiency are asymptomatic and do not develop recurrent infections. Screening of these patients has revealed that approximately 10 percent have CD; conversely, 1 to 2 percent of all individuals with CD have selective IgA deficiency. Selective IgA deficiency can complicate making the diagnosis of CD, because all of the blood testing for CD is based on IgA antibody blood testing. If a person does not make **immunoglobulin A (IgA),** then he or she cannot have a positive blood test even in the presence of the disease. In such cases, alternative blood testing is required for diagnosis.

Associated Diseases

Type 1 diabetes (juvenile diabetes) starts in childhood and is not associated with obesity. This autoimmune disease affects the pancreas, destroying the cells that make insulin. It is treated with lifelong insulin shots. Type 2 diabetes (adult-onset diabetes) is much more common in the United States, in part because it is associated with obesity; in this condition, the body becomes less responsive to normal insulin production. Studies show that 2.6 to 7.8 percent of children with type 1 diabetes have CD. The disease association is complicated, however, in that both type 1 diabetes and CD are autoimmune diseases and both are associated with the gene for HLA-DQ2.

Dermatitis herpetiformis (DH) is very strongly associated with CD (it is covered in more detail in Part 7 of this book). This intensely itchy rash is characterized by tiny blisters that occur on the extremities and trunk. Diagnosis is made by skin biopsy, checking for abnormal skin IgA antibody deposits. More than 85 percent of patients with DH have CD, and as many as 24 percent of patients with CD have DH.

A variety of other autoimmune diseases are also associated with an increased risk of CD—namely, thyroid disease, liver disease, vitiligo, and **Sjogren's syndrome** (dry eyes and mouth).

Official recommendations of the North American Society for Pediatric Gastroenterology, Hepatology, and Nutrition are

that children and adolescents with symptoms of celiac disease or an increased risk for celiac disease have a blood test for antibody to tissue transglutaminase (tTG), that those with an elevated tTG be referred to a pediatric gastroenterologist for an intestinal biopsy,

Immunoglobulin A (IgA)

A type of immunoglobulin that is used to test for celiac disease. It is absent in individuals with selective IgA deficiency.

Type 1 diabetes

An autoimmune disease of the pancreas that affects children. It is often associated with celiac disease.

Sjogren's syndrome

An autoimmune disease of the tear glands and salivary glands that results in dry eyes and mouth.

Children and Celiac Disease

and that those with the characteristics of celiac disease on intestinal histopathology be treated with a strict gluten-free diet.

A recent National Institutes of Health consensus conference on CD was less emphatic and recommends that testing be considered for children at increased risk, particularly those with symptoms.

30. Is there a link between celiac disease and autism?

Autism

A disorder beginning at an early age that is characterized by delays or difficulty with communication, language, and social interaction.

Autism is a common developmental disorder, with recent studies suggesting that it affects 1 in every 166 children in the United States. Autism generally first appears in early childhood and is characterized by impaired social interaction and communication with absent speech in approximately 50 percent of children. Autistic children may exhibit a variety of abnormal behaviors, including resistance to change and repetitive movements such as hand flapping and body rocking. The cause of autism is unknown, although some researchers believe that there may be a genetic component. This suspicion is based on the high rate of autism in identical twins, though the fact that most identical twins are raised in the same environment may be a causative factor.

One study of autistic children that focused on the presence of gastrointestinal disease found that these children have a high risk of gastroesophageal reflux disease, inflammation of the stomach and duodenum, low intestinal digestive enzyme levels, and an underactive pancreas that responds to the hormone **secretin.** The same investigators showed that the patients' autistic symptoms improved after treatment with secretin shots. However, several subsequent studies did not confirm the benefit of secretin therapy in autism.

Secretin

A synthetic hormone used in gastrointestinal testing that has variable benefits for autism.

Multiple studies have failed to show a direct, conclusive link between CD and autism. Children with autism have been tested for CD, and children with CD have been tested for autism; even so, most studies do not demonstrate an increased risk for having both conditions simultaneously. One hypothesis suggests that autistic children have a **leaky gut** (increased gut permeability), which might increase their risk for developing CD. The gut is a barrier that generally lets things into the body selectively, thereby controlling these materials' access to other parts of the body. The "leaky gut" hypothesis suggests that in autism the gut allows small molecules into the circulation, which may in turn stimulate the brain. This controversial idea has not been confirmed by medical studies, but it is intriguing given the role of the leaky gut in CD and potential therapies (see Question 57).

Because of the leaky gut theory, several studies have examined the effects of a gluten-free diet on children with autism. Some behavioral improvements have also been reported in autistic children who followed a **gluten-free** and **casein-free diet.** Casein is a protein from milk that is commonly used to supplement food. These studies on the effects of a restrictive diet on autism have yielded mixed results, however, and some have not demonstrated any benefit.

31. Should my children be checked for celiac disease?

A 2005 article in the medical journal *Gastroenterology* discussed the issue of screening children for CD and provided some guidelines. These guidelines were based on the available medical literature and took several factors into account:

- What is the severity of the disease? (That is, is there any benefit to diagnosing children without any symptoms?)
- Will children who test positive for CD be willing to go on a gluten-free diet?
- Does a gluten-free diet benefit asymptomatic people and those with potential CD?
- Are the screening methods sensitive and specific enough to minimize false-positive and false-negative results?

Leaky gut

Inflammation of the intestine that promotes leakiness of the gut lining, thereby allowing foreign proteins in.

Gluten-free diet

A diet completely free of any gluten.

Casein-free diet

Casein is a protein derived from milk. A casein-free and gluten-free diet is sometimes suggested for patients with autism.

Children and Celiac Disease

Screening of all children for CD is currently not recommended. Based on the frequency of CD in the general population (approximately 1 in 100 people), individuals who are deemed to be at higher risk should be screened. In particular, children with Down syndrome, Williams syndrome, Turner syndrome, and selective IgA deficiency should be screened. Children with type 1 diabetes, thyroid disease, autoimmune liver disease, anemia, short stature, delayed puberty, dermatitis herpetiformis, recurrent oral ulcers, dental abnormalities, and malnutrition should be tested as well. Symptoms of abdominal bloating, chronic diarrhea, constipation, vomiting, failure to thrive, and irritability may warrant evaluation. First-degree relatives should also be tested, particularly if they have symptoms.

Table 9   Rates of Celiac Disease in High-Risk Populations

General U.S.	1 in 100
Type 1 Diabetes	1 in 25
First-degree relative	1 in 10
Autoimmune thyroid disease	1 in 33
Down, Williams, Turner syndrome	1 in 10
IgA Deficiency	1 in 50
Dermatitis herpetiformis	over 90%

These recommendations are based on science and apply to populations rather than specific individuals. If you are the one who gets the disease, the risk of CD is 100 percent for you, not 1 in 100. I am not a pediatrician and do not take care of children, but I am a father, so I will not make a recommendation regarding testing of pediatric patients, just a suggestion. Clearly, CD has many manifestations. Given the ease with which screening can be done, I have a very low threshold for checking my adult patients for this disease.

32. How is celiac disease diagnosed in children? Should my child see a specialist?

Testing for diagnosis of CD in children is the same as it is in adults. Initial testing of those at risk consists of blood tests for the antiendomysial antibody (EMA), or the tissue trans-glutaminase antibody (tTG). If these tests are positive, then an endoscopy needs to be done to obtain a biopsy of the small intestine. Visual examination of the duodenal lining may show atrophy, a mosaic pattern, scalloping, redness, and irritation; however, these findings by themselves are insufficient to make the diagnosis. If the biopsy shows variable amounts of blunting or atrophy of the villi with increased inflammatory cells, then the diagnosis is confirmed.

The biopsy is the "gold standard" for diagnosis in both children and adults. The biopsy in conjunction with blood testing is required for definitive diagnosis, as other processes may potentially result in a similar biopsy. For example, a bad intestinal bug or flu, bacterial overgrowth, and tropical sprue are just a few conditions that can mimic CD on biopsy.

A variant on this case is the child with latent or potential CD who has a positive blood test with a normal biopsy. Such a child might have CD—sometimes the distribution of the intestinal inflammation is patchy, so it may be missed on endoscopy. Alternatively, the child truly may have latent disease and develop CD in the future; in such a case, the child should be monitored to see whether symptoms appear.

Another variant is the child with a selective IgA deficiency. Children with this condition do not produce IgA and will have negative blood tests even in the presence of CD. Blood testing for IgG antibodies to AGA, EMA, or tTG is required in such a scenario and usually requires a special request by your healthcare provider. In case of selective IgA deficiency, the biopsy will show the appropriate inflammatory changes if CD is present.

Finally, to get positive blood testing or small intestine biopsies, the child must be on a gluten-containing diet prior to testing. For more information on the diagnosis of CD, see Part 4 of this book.

I would recommend taking your child to a specialist (such as a pediatric gastroenterologist) at least to make the appropriate diagnosis. Endoscopic testing on children should be done by someone with experience who performs these procedures regularly, as there is a major difference between doing endoscopy in children and adults. Adults usually receive "conscious sedation," which means that they are sedated but conscious and can follow instructions. Children usually receive general anesthesia because they cannot cooperate with the exam and to provide comfort and amnesia. This deeper level of sedation is usually provided by an anesthesiologist.

The official recommendation of the North American Society for Pediatric Gastroenterology, Hepatology, and Nutrition is that children with symptoms of CD or an increased risk of this disease should have a blood test for the antibody to tTG. If the tTG test is positive, the child should be referred to a pediatric gastroenterologist for an endoscopy and intestinal biopsy.

33. What is the treatment for celiac disease in children?

Treatment for children and adolescents with CD is a gluten-free diet. The caveat is that children with potential or latent disease should probably not be given a gluten-free diet. There is some debate over this point, however, so you should check with your pediatrician.

Of course, the process and issues are different for children who must follow such a diet than the process and issues for adult patients. Young children will likely do the best, as they will eat a gluten-free diet and not miss "regular" food.

They do not understand that they have a chronic illness that requires lifelong adherence to a restricted diet. The elementary school years can be difficult, as children face teasing that they are different, and peer pressure can make dietary compliance difficult. The adolescent years are likely the most difficult owing to puberty and the great social pressures faced by youths. Members of this age group are trying to establish independence and define themselves, fostering at least some rebellion. Weight is also an issue with adolescents, and many are at risk for eating disorders and obesity.

Children-oriented support groups and some authors have recommended a variety of strategies to help parents and children work together to stay gluten free. Teaching good dietary habits at a young age will result in good long-term habits. Children need to take responsibility for their disease and be empowered. They need to read labels and help prepare their own menus and food. They need to understand their food allergy and be able to educate friends, teachers, daycare providers, and relatives about CD. Support groups are an important resource for children for educational purposes, reinforcing diet compliance and offering an opportunity to meet other children with CD. It is important to know that you are not the only one with a chronic disease, and having friends with similar issues both is supportive and can be an emotional outlet. In addition, children need to be in a safe environment at school; teachers, the school nurse, and food providers need to be made aware of their dietary sensitivities and restrictions.

The gluten-free diet is the same for both children and adults, so they share many common issues, including sources of contamination and non-dietary gluten. Please see the various questions on the gluten-free diet elsewhere in this book; Question 98 deals specifically with resources for children.

Children should take gluten-free vitamin and mineral supplements and be assessed for any deficiencies; if any are found, the deficiencies should be corrected. You and your child should be referred to a pediatric dietitian for dietary instruction, gluten-free teaching, recommendation of supplements, and educational material. Most importantly, follow-up appointments are required to check for dietary compliance and to address ongoing questions and issues. Follow-up with a physician is required to ensure proper growth, weight gain, and correction of deficiencies. Joining your local children's CD support group can be a helpful resource for both you and your child.

34. What are the complications of celiac disease in children?

Both adults and children may experience long-term complications of CD. Although these complications are mostly the same for both age groups, some are unique to children. In particular, symptoms and chronic discomfort in children can have effects on personality development, difficulty in school, self-image, and feelings about healthy weight. Small children can have failure to thrive, which leads to poor muscle tone, poor weight gain, and pale, frail, underweight, and small-for-size stature.

Normal growth requires adequate nutrition, including appropriate amounts of protein, vitamin D, calcium, and phosphorus to promote healthy bones. Celiac disease impairs vitamin D and calcium absorption, thereby stunting bone growth and resulting in short stature. Vitamin D malabsorption can cause rickets, osteopenia, and osteoporosis, all of which are associated with low **bone mineral density (BMD)**. A study that compared 44 Italian children with CD to normal controls found significantly lower BMD in children with untreated CD. After one year on a gluten-free diet, however, the BMD in the CD group returned to normal.

Bone mineral density (BMD)

A measure of the mineral content (a marker for osteoporosis).

Calcium and vitamin D are involved in the production of tooth enamel (the hard white outer layer of the tooth). Children with CD who have abnormal enamel production can develop discolored teeth that are prone to cavities. **Aphthous mouth ulcers** are a mouth symptom associated with CD. Low vitamin D levels can also cause muscle weakness and twitching as well as an overactive **parathyroid gland.**

Because children are growing, they have increased requirements for nutrients and vitamins. This greater demand, in turn, places them at increased risk for deficiency. Deficiencies of several nutrients, vitamins, and minerals other than vitamin D and calcium are common in children with CD. For example, anemia is noted in approximately 4 percent of all patients newly diagnosed with CD. Anemia in children may be multifactorial in origin, deriving from chronic illness and deficiencies of iron, folic acid, and vitamin B_{12}. **Zinc** deficiency is common in diarrheal illness and is clinically manifested as rash, poor wound healing, and an altered sense of taste. Magnesium is a poorly absorbed mineral, but its supplementation may worsen GI symptoms, thereby exacerbating diarrhea. Low magnesium levels can cause muscle cramping and irregular heart rates. Delayed puberty is another potential sign of vitamin deficits: Recent studies suggest that low dietary intake or malabsorption of B vitamins, folic acid, and iron may contribute to delayed puberty. Unlike gluten-free products, most wheat products are enriched with essential vitamins; this difference can further exacerbate deficiencies in patients with CD who follow a gluten-free diet.

There is a strong association between type 1 diabetes and CD, such that 4 percent of people who have diabetes also have CD. Control of diabetes relies on several measures: a prescribed diet that avoids high-sugar foods, reliable food absorption, insulin shots, and frequent blood sugar testing. If sugars are not controlled over the long term, then the risk of complications of diabetes—for example, vascular and heart disease, **neuropathy** (numbness and tingling in the hands and feet), blindness, and kidney disease—increases. The challenges faced by a child with both diabetes and CD are great, given the chronic illness, need for insulin shots, blood sugar testing

---

Children and Celiac Disease

Aphthous mouth ulcers

Recurrent sores or ulcers in the mouth that may be associated with celiac disease.

Parathyroid gland

A gland located in the neck that produces parathyroid hormone.

Zinc

An essential mineral that maintains the body's wound-healing ability.

Neuropathy

An inflammatory condition of nerves that is accompanied by numbness and tingling of the arms and legs.

Table 10   Nutrients That May Be Deficient in Children with Celiac Disease

Nutrient	Normal Role
Vitamin A	Healthy vision
Vitamin D	Bone growth and formation
B vitamins	Nervous system function, blood formation, sexual development
Calcium	Bone growth and muscle function
Iron	Blood production
Magnesium	Muscle and heart function
Zinc	Wound healing, taste function and skin integrity
Fiber	Normal bowel function

many times each day, and strict diet possibly compounded with the addition of a gluten restriction. For these children, a gluten-free diet will improve food and nutrient absorption, stabilizing blood sugar control and minimizing the risk of complications from both the diabetes and the CD.

Neurologic complications of CD may affect both children and adults. Neurologic manifestations in children with CD may include **hypotonia** (muscle weakness), paralysis, chronic headache, developmental delay, learning disabilities, ataxia (difficulty walking), seizures, depression, and possibly attention-deficient hyperactivity disorder. Some of these entities may improve if a gluten-free diet is implemented early on. As discussed in Question 30, there does not appear to be a strong link between autism and CD, but there may be a behavioral benefit for children with autism who follow a gluten-free diet.

Celiac disease also increases a child's risk of developing other autoimmune diseases, such as thyroid, liver, and skin disease. Periodic testing of thyroid and liver functions is required for detection of these conditions. An overactive or underactive thyroid must be treated to ensure normal growth, permit

Hypotonia

Muscle weakness; the "floppiness" seen in a child.

appropriate weight gain, and prevent complications. Children with CD are at increased risk for abnormal liver tests, chronic hepatitis, fatty liver disease, cirrhosis of the liver, primary biliary cirrhosis, and sclerosing cholangitis. All of these conditions need to be diagnosed early to prevent or minimize progressive liver damage.

Study results are mixed but suggest that children have an increased risk of obesity after initiation of a gluten-free diet. This diet promotes healing of the damaged small intestine and improves digestion and absorption of nutrients, leading to a net gain in calories absorbed. Gluten products are carbohydrates and starches, so eliminating them results in a dietary imbalance that favors absorption of a higher percentage of calories as fats. One study of celiac adolescents on a gluten-free diet found that the rate of overweight or obesity in those adolescents who complied with a strict diet was 72 percent; in children not following a strict diet, 51 percent were overweight or obese, compared to 47 percent of healthy controls.

The issues of increased cancer risk and mortality associated with CD have not adequately been addressed in children. Certainly, the adult data demonstrate the benefit of a gluten-free diet in minimizing these extreme celiac complications.

Overall, the gluten-free diet offers a substantial benefit in children. Nutritional deficiencies of calories, protein, vitamins, minerals, and fiber can be corrected, improving the child's well-being and decreasing his or her risk of complications. This outcome is very compelling with respect to bone disease, weight issues at diagnosis, diabetic control, and neurologic disease. Of course, a gluten-free diet is a lifelong endeavor, because children with CD become adults with CD. The earlier good gluten-free dietary habits can be established, the better the ultimate result. A pediatric dietitian will be a valuable partner for you and your family and can help with this process. Regular visits to healthcare professionals are also needed to prevent excessive weight gain and childhood obesity.

PART FOUR

Evaluation and Diagnosis

How is celiac disease diagnosed?

Do I need to see a specialist?

What are the blood tests for celiac disease?

More...

Antigliadin antibody (AGA)

An IgA antibody blood test that is fairly sensitive for detection of celiac disease. It can also produce false positive and negative results.

Antiendomysial antibody (EMA)

A sensitive blood test commonly used to test for celiac disease. The EMA is an IgA antibody test.

Tissue transglutaminase antibody (tTG)

A blood test commonly used to screen for celiac disease.

If any or all of the blood test results are positive, they suggest the diagnosis of CD but do not definitively prove the disease's presence. The "gold standard" for diagnosis of CD remains a small bowel biopsy.

35. How is celiac disease diagnosed?

The diagnosis of CD has evolved over the years thanks to improvements in blood tests and greater ease in performing endoscopy and obtaining biopsies. Individuals without symptoms, such as family members of someone with diagnosed CD and patients with unexplained anemia, osteoporosis, or increased liver tests, can now be screened for CD with blood tests. Patients who are symptomatic can also undergo blood testing, although sometimes they are directly referred for endoscopy and small intestine biopsies prior to the blood tests.

Several blood tests are used to support the diagnosis of CD, and some are better than others at identifying the disease. The typical tests are **antigliadin antibody (AGA), antiendomysial antibody (EMA),** and **tissue transglutaminase antibody (tTG)**. The widespread use of these tests has revealed that CD is actually fairly common: In the U.S. population, the tests are positive in about 1 in 100 people. These blood tests require an order by your doctor or healthcare provider; they cannot be requested directly by a patient. They involve a single blood draw, and results are usually available in a week. If any or all of the test results are positive, they suggest the diagnosis of CD but do not definitively prove the disease's presence. The "gold standard" for diagnosis of CD remains a small bowel biopsy.

Biopsies of the small intestine mucosa can show inflammation and abnormalities in the villi. These finger-like projections increase the surface area of the small intestine, maximizing contact between the nutrient-rich fluid and the gut. Thus the villi are the site of breakdown of food products and their subsequent absorption into the bloodstream. In CD, the villi can be shortened, atrophied, or completely destroyed by inflammation. Examination of biopsies under the microscope may demonstrate normal or healthy villi or the changes seen in CD. This evaluation can also help determine whether another disease is present and rule out a disease whose symptoms mimic those of CD.

Celiac disease is not diagnosed with a trial of a gluten-free diet. Likewise, it is not diagnosed with skin allergy testing. Blood testing and endoscopy are required for accurate diagnosis. Many medical practitioners, including alternative or holistic practitioners, may make a diagnosis based on the patient's response to withdrawal of gluten products from the diet. This assumption is often incorrect, however, because gluten is a complex dietary protein that is difficult to break down and absorb. Many patients may experience improved symptoms with a gluten-free diet yet not have CD. For example, they may actually have gluten sensitivity or IBS that responds to a gluten restriction.

Celiac disease is not diagnosed with a trial of a gluten-free diet, nor is it diagnosed with skin allergy testing.

Although CD sounds like a simple diagnosis to make, sometimes it can be difficult to determine whether a patient actually has the disease. A biopsy may be positive with negative blood testing, or blood testing may be positive with a negative biopsy. Some blood tests are nonspecific, meaning that a positive test does not always equal disease. Approximately 5 percent of patients with CD have selective IgA deficiency; these individuals do not have the capacity to produce certain antibodies and, therefore, have false-negative results with the standard blood tests. Luckily, most patients with CD have positive blood tests and biopsies confirming the diagnosis.

36. Do I need to see a specialist?

The short answer is yes. Because of the previously mentioned confusion in diagnosis, a specialist can help clarify whether you really have CD. Gastroenterologists are doctors who have completed training in general medicine and have undergone several years of additional training in diseases of the gut, liver, and pancreas. Most gastroenterologists perform procedures such as upper endoscopy, in which a scope or other instrument is passed into the mouth of a sedated patient and down

Evaluation and Diagnosis

the esophagus, stomach, and duodenum. Various tools can be passed down the scope for tissue sampling or management of bleeding. Generally, a gastroenterologist performs the endoscopic biopsy confirming the diagnosis of CD.

Gastroenterologists treat, diagnose, and manage CD, much in the same way that cardiologists (heart doctors) treat patients who have suffered a heart attack. Gastroenterologists understand the various blood tests used to make the diagnosis of CD, are aware of the diseases that mimic CD, and can sort out the issues. Further, they know the complications of CD and can help you manage them.

Depending on where you live and which types of specialists are available, some gastroenterologists may have an interest or subspecialty in diseases of the small intestine such as CD (like me). These doctors usually practice or are affiliated with larger hospitals or teaching institutions that train other doctors. They generally take on the more difficult or confusing cases that have been referred by the local gastroenterologist for further evaluation and management.

Marye comments:

I strongly believe that you should see a specialist for celiac disease. In talking to people with celiac disease, many had to force their doctors to give them the blood test for this disease. Several people found out that they had celiac disease by searching for their symptoms online.

37. Should I be checked for celiac disease?

Patients with gastrointestinal symptoms who have lactose intolerance or those diagnosed with IBS should definitely be checked for CD. Obviously, individuals with chronic diarrhea, abdominal symptoms, and vitamin deficiencies should be evaluated for this disease as well. These kinds of symptoms accompanied by unexplained weight loss are a "red flag" that warrant a doctor's visit. Testing for CD is strongly recommended as part of a medical evaluation for explained weight loss.

Celiac disease is an autoimmune disease, and those patients with other autoimmune diseases such as vitiligo (white patches of skin), lupus, **rheumatoid arthritis,** and thyroid disease are at higher risk for developing it. In such cases, CD can be silent or have atypical symptoms. Depression or psychiatric illness, thyroid abnormalities, fertility issues, osteoporosis, and type 1 diabetes may all be extra-intestinal manifestations of CD. Patients with **iron-deficiency anemia, pernicious anemia** (low vitamin B_{12} level), or osteoporosis with low vitamin D levels may also have CD.

Asymptomatic family members of a person with CD have a 10 percent chance of developing CD, so screening blood tests should be considered for these individuals. The children and siblings of persons with CD should probably be screened as well, and even second- or third-degree relatives may be affected. Population-based studies in the United States suggest that about 1 in 100 people has CD. If you are of Irish, Italian, or French Canadian ancestry, your risk may even be higher.

Dermatitis herpetiformis (DH) is a skin rash that is intensely itchy, with tiny blisters appearing on the arms and trunk. Nevertheless, this condition is difficult to diagnose because the blisters are usually scratched away by the time patients reach the physician's office. Instead, the diagnosis of DH is typically made by biopsy of the skin. Virtually all patients with DH have CD, but only a small proportion of patients with CD have DH. All patients with DH should undergo testing for CD, including a small intestinal biopsy.

Screening for CD is easy and involves a single blood test ordered by your doctor. You should discuss with your doctor whether testing is indicated in your particular circumstances. If the test results are positive, further evaluation will be needed

Rheumatoid arthritis

An autoimmune arthritis that causes joint inflammation and destruction.

Iron-deficiency anemia

A type of anemia caused by depleted iron stores.

Pernicious anemia

A vitamin B_{12} deficiency that results in anemia.

Evaluation and Diagnosis

and an appointment with a specialist (a gastroenterologist) is recommended. In particular, more blood testing and an endoscopy may be required to confirm the diagnosis.

38. What are the blood tests for celiac disease?

First, a brief education on the immune system is in order. Your immune system protects you from infections and helps to heal wounds. If the immune system is overactive, it can result in autoimmune diseases such as lupus, vitiligo, rheumatoid arthritis, and CD. Celiac disease is an autoimmune process, meaning that the body attacks itself or something that the body recognizes as foreign. In the case of CD, gluten stimulates the immune system to clear or destroy the lining of the small intestine. The immune system "thinks" that the gut lining is a foreign invader like a bacteria or virus.

The immune system is extremely complicated and has many parts; among them are the cellular and the humoral components. The **cellular immune system** comprises many different types of cells that work together, "communicating" to fight infection. One type of cell may identify things as foreign, another type of cell may recruit other cells to move to a particular area or organ, and a third type of cell may actually kill the bacteria.

The other major part of the immune system is the **humoral immune system**. It includes cells that make antibodies, which are proteins that circulate in the bloodstream and bind to foreign proteins. When bound to a foreign protein, antibodies stimulate the immune system to attack the protein, thereby protecting the body from infection. An example of this activity can be seen with a flu shot, in which foreign proteins that are normally found on the surface of the flu virus are injected into your arm. These proteins circulate throughout the body and are "seen" by the humoral immune system, which responds by producing antibodies specific to the flu protein. Later, when you are exposed to the flu by a sneezing colleague at work, the

Cellular immune system

One of the two major parts of the immune system, along with the humoral immune system. The cellular immune system is where various immune cells locate, attract, and destroy bacteria or viruses.

Humoral immune system

One of the two major parts of the immune system. It makes the immunoglobulins that fight infection.

Three antibody tests commonly done when diagnosing CD, which detect antigliadin antibody (AGA), antiendomysial antibody (EMA), and tissue transglutaminase antibody (tTG), respectively.

virus enters your body and the antibodies react by coating the virus and killing it, protecting you from infection.

This process is somewhat complicated, but an explanation of immunity is required to really understand how CD is diagnosed. Most of the blood tests for CD detect abnormal antibodies in the bloodstream. Three antibody tests are commonly done, which detect antigliadin antibody (AGA), antiendomysial antibody (EMA), and tissue transglutaminase antibody (tTG), respectively. Some laboratories offer a group of tests called a "celiac panel" that the doctor might order; alternatively, a single test might be performed to screen for CD. The AGA, EMA, and tTG tests are not identical, and some are definitely better than others at identifying CD. Further, if a celiac panel is done, some tests may be positive while others are negative, adding great confusion to the picture.

39. What is the recommended blood testing for celiac disease?

The keys to understanding whether a particular test is a good option for diagnosing are the concepts of sensitivity and specificity. **Sensitivity** is the ability of a test to pick up true-positive results, in which case the person really does have CD; **specificity** is the ability to identify whether a negative result really means that the person does not have the disease.

Sensitivity
The ability of a test to detect a true positive result.

Specificity
The ability of a test to pick up a true positive result.

Table 11 Understanding the Sensitivity and Specificity of Blood Tests

	Patient with CD	Patient without CD
Positive test	True Positives	False Positives
Negative test	False Negatives	True Negatives
	Sensitivity	**Specificity**

Table 11 may help to clarify these confusing concepts. These issues are important in that some CD tests are very sensitive, meaning that they will identify most patients with CD. Other tests are not specific, meaning that a positive test may or may not truly identify CD, leading to false-positive diagnoses. Thus the goal of testing is a test that is both highly specific and highly sensitive for detection of CD.

Common to all CD blood tests is the use of a single needle stick or blood draw to collect the sample. These tests are widely commercially available and are performed in a fairly standardized manner by most laboratories. Results are generally available in about a week. Such testing may help diagnose any type of CD regardless of whether the patient has symptoms, is an asymptomatic child of someone with confirmed CD, or has atypical manifestations of the disease. Although the tests can suggest CD, they are not the "gold standard" for diagnosis. Instead, a small bowel biopsy is recommended for confirmation of CD.

The antiendomysial antibody (EMA) is a complicated test in which the patient's blood is processed, placed on a glass slide containing one of several types of tissues, and observed to see whether antibodies in the blood will bind to the tissue in a certain pattern. For the EMA, the tissue used is either monkey esophagus tissue or human umbilical cord tissue. The problem with the former option is that it requires monkeys to be killed and their esophagi removed for processing. This raises ethical issues, is very expensive and difficult to do, and requires a lot of monkeys. By contrast, human umbilical cords are generally considered a waste product of birth and are easier to obtain. Nevertheless, because of these issues and complexity of completing this test, the EMA is falling out of favor (although it is still commonly used and widely available today).

The EMA is a highly reliable test for diagnosis of CD and has been used as a screening test for this disease for many years.

The EMA is a highly reliable test for diagnosis of CD and has been used as a screening test for this disease for many years. Either type of EMA (monkey esophagus tissue or human umbilical cord tissue) is very sensitive for both adults and children with CD, identifying more than 90 percent of cases correctly. In some studies, its accuracy approaches nearly 100 percent. The EMA's specificity for both adults and children is high, exceeding 95 percent in most studies.

Tissue transglutaminase (tTG) antibody is a fairly new test for CD and has been evolving over the last few years to become easier to perform. Most commercial labs currently use human engineered red blood cell proteins as a substrate for this test. This approach is beneficial in that nothing is harmed during production of the test and an unlimited supply of tests is available. In adults and children, the sensitivity of the tTG exceeds 95 percent in terms of its ability to identify CD successfully. Specificity for the tTG for both groups is more than 98 percent, nearly eliminating any false-positive tests.

The oldest blood test for CD is the antigliadin antibody (AGA) test. The AGA has been around for decades and has evolved and improved over time. It is currently part of the celiac panel of tests. The AGA is fairly sensitive, successfully identifying more than 85 percent of CD cases. Its specificity ranges from 85 percent to 90 percent, meaning that the AGA can produce false-positive results, leading to confusion in the initial diagnosis. There may be a role for AGA testing in other circumstances, such as follow-up care or confirmation of CD.

Table 12   The Sensitivity and Specificity of Commonly Available Antibody Blood Tests for Celiac Disease

Test	Sensitivity	Specificity	Recommend for Screening
Antiendomysial Antibody (EMA)	90 to 100%	>95%	Yes
Tissue Transglutaminase Antibody (tTG)	>95%	>98%	Yes
Antigliadin Antibody (AGA)	>85%	85 to 90%	No

In my practice, when screening for CD among family members and patients with GI or atypical symptoms, I recommend an EMA or tTG. I order tTG tests for my patients. Sometimes, if a doctor orders an EMA, the lab will automatically change it to a tTG, as both are very reliable tests. At this time, I would not recommend an AGA test for screening, because better tests are available that avoid the potential for false-positive results.

I do not order celiac panel testing. This group of tests may be helpful for doctors who do not usually treat CD and do not understand the intricacies of testing, however. Panel testing, if it yields all-positive or all-negative results, quickly resolves the diagnosis. If it produces mixed results, by contrast, the outcome may be confusion. Suppose the results include a negative EMA and tTG but a positive AGA. Does the patient have CD? Well, you cannot make the diagnosis either way. Confirmatory testing and possibly endoscopy will be needed for definitive diagnosis in such cases.

40. What are the pitfalls or problems with blood testing for celiac disease?

For most patients, the actual blood testing process is straightforward. By comparison, the results of such testing can be ambiguous, be confusing, and lead to incorrect diagnoses for patients. Physicians who do not regularly treat patients with CD may not understand the nuances associated with testing. In my practice, I see many patients who are referred by other doctors for CD, and I rule out this diagnosis almost as often as I confirm it. Misdiagnosis may lead to an unnecessary, possibly lifelong gluten-free diet with its associated cost, inconvenience, and stigma. Misdiagnosis also labels patients, leads to extra medical testing and doctor visits, and generates unneeded worry about complications such as cancer. Thus the first major problem with blood testing for CD is inappropriate physician interpretation of the results.

Another shortcoming of blood testing is the inconsistency of results (see Question 39). The tests for CD are not perfect: Some produce false-positive and false-negative results. If re-testing is ordered, results may change for the same patient. Many labs report the result of antibody testing as a number within a range from negative to indeterminate to positive. If your test result is indeterminate, what does that mean? If you are high normal or low positive, what is the significance? A wise colleague once told me, if you have vague gastrointestinal symptoms, "it could be early something or late nothing." I generally suggest repeat testing or running a different test to narrow the diagnosis if the initial picture is unclear.

As mentioned earlier, management of CD relies on a gluten-free diet. This diet improves symptoms and resolves the inflammation and damage seen in small intestine biopsies. A strict gluten-free diet will make previously positive blood test results become negative. This is beneficial because it is a good way to follow CD over time. If screening is done while a patient is on a gluten-free diet, however, the tests can be negative, thereby hiding the presence of CD. For this reason, it is key that all initial testing—both blood tests and small bowel biopsies—be done while the patient is on a gluten-containing diet.

Question 38 introduced the immune system. Blood testing for CD focuses on the humoral immune system and its production of antibodies. Although the body manufactures many different kinds of antibodies, the main types are **immuno-globulins**—specifically, immunoglobulins A (IgA), D (IgD), E (IgE), G (IgG), and M (IgM). Celiac blood tests, including the EMA, tTG, and AGA, all assess IgA levels.

One of the most commonly encountered defects or abnormalities in the immune system is selective IgA deficiency, in which the body does not manufacture IgA. Selective IgA deficiency is 10 to 15 times more common in people with

A strict gluten-free diet will make previously positive blood test results become negative. For this reason, it is key that all initial testing—both blood tests and small bowel biopsies—be done while the patient is on a gluten-containing diet.

Immunoglobulin

A bodily protein that fights infection and mediates inflammation.

Evaluation and Diagnosis

CD compared to the general population. Indeed, as many as 8 percent of all patients with CD have selective IgA deficiency. As children, individuals with this deficiency are predisposed to ear infections, bronchitis, and sinus infections, which can persist into adulthood. Because patients with CD and selective IgA deficiency cannot make the IgA antibodies to EMA, tTG, and AGA, all of these tests will be negative despite the presence of CD.

If there is a high suspicion for CD but testing is negative, then the doctor may check the patient's IgA level. This test will reveal whether the individual has an IgA deficiency and if they can make IgA antibodies. Of course, it still does not confirm the presence or absence of CD. If the patient does have an IgA deficiency, then the "usual" CD blood tests will produce

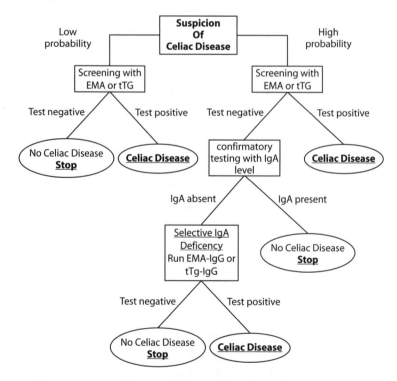

Figure 5 **An algorithm for celiac blood testing. All positive blood test results must be confirmed with endoscopic small intestine biopsies.**

false-negative results, and special tests are needed. Antibody tests for EMA, tTG, and AGA are all available as IgG tests if the physician makes a special request to the laboratory.

The most difficult and confusing group when trying to diagnose CD is patients with CD who have no positive tests. A small percentage of patients with CD are "antibody negative" for all tests. Question 41 offers an expanded discussion of this subgroup.

41. Can I have celiac disease even though my blood test results are negative?

The answer to this question is yes, but such a scenario is incredibly rare and probably accounts for fewer than 1 percent of those patients with CD. These patients with negative antibody tests do not have a selective IgA deficiency and should have the capacity to make antibodies. This is a curious situation in that all test results—the EMA, tTG, and AGA for both IgA and IgG antibodies—are negative. It makes diagnosis of CD very difficult, such that these patients often face a long illness with misdiagnosis or delayed diagnosis. In such cases, the definitive diagnosis is usually made when the patient experiences weight loss or a vitamin deficiency that prompts an endoscopy and small bowel biopsy, where the results suggest CD. Antibody-negative patients will have CD symptoms and small intestine biopsies consistent with CD. These patients respond to a gluten-free diet and are said to have true CD despite no supporting blood tests.

The path to diagnosis for antibody-negative patients does not conform to the flowchart presented in Question 40 (Figure 5). Indeed, if the patient seeks medical attention and is asymptomatic or demonstrates atypical symptoms, the correct diagnosis may never be made. Generally, these patients receive a correct diagnosis after evaluation by a specialist in treating celiac patients. In my practice, I have made this diagnosis once—after a chronically ill patient with diarrhea, weight loss, and multiple vitamin deficiencies was referred by another gastroenterologist after years of evading an appropriate diagnosis. In this case, endoscopy and biopsy revealed the classic changes consistent with CD. After a year on a gluten-free diet, this patient regained all of her weight, and all of her symptoms and vitamin deficiencies resolved.

A word of caution: Many patients who seek medical attention may have diarrhea and other nonspecific symptoms. Screening with an EMA or tTG is enough to exclude CD in most such patients. On rare occasions, if the suspicion for CD is high, then an IgA level or IgG antibody testing can be done. These tests are sufficient to exclude CD in more than 99 percent of all patients. Gluten sensitivity is much more common than antibody-negative CD, and it really requires evaluation by a specialist for correct diagnosis.

42. Is the antigliadin antibody useful?

The AGA was the first blood screening test for CD and has been available for decades. It is fairly sensitive and specific for picking up true CD. Nevertheless, better tests are just as readily available, so the general recommendation is that the AGA not be used for CD screening. The AGA misses 10 to 15 percent of CD cases and gives a false-positive result in 10 percent of cases. This failure can either delay or miss the diagnosis, so that the patient goes without treatment, or unnecessarily suggest the presence of CD, so that the patient begins an inappropriate diet or undergoes invasive testing to rule out the diagnosis. For these reasons, in my practice I do not order the AGA or any celiac panel of tests that include the AGA.

The AGA might play a role for patients with ambiguous test results, for patients with selective IgA deficiency, or in the evaluation of antibody-negative patients. I rarely request AGA testing, though I may use it as a backup test, particularly in patients who have a high likelihood of having CD but

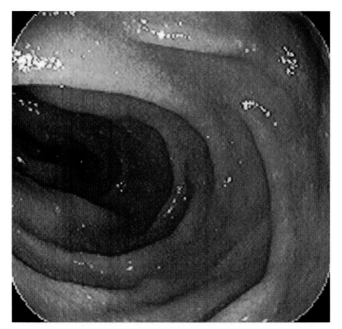

Color Plate 1   Endoscopic photo of normal duodenum.

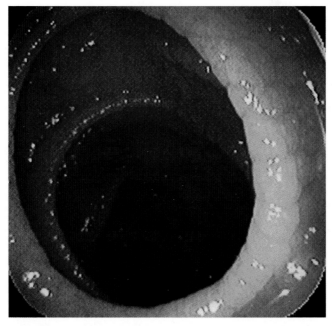

Color Plate 2   Endoscopic photo of duodenum in a patient with celiac disease.

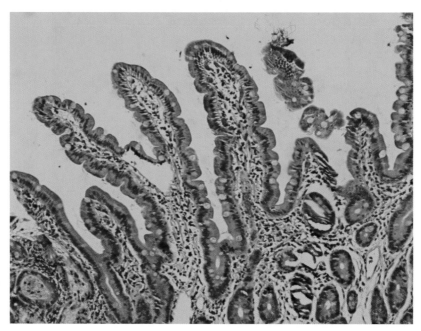

Color Plate 3   Microscopic color photo of normal duodenum lining.

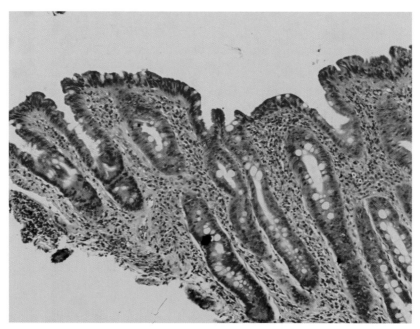

Color Plate 4   Microscopic color photo of celiac disease a Marsh level IIIc lesion with absent villi and elongated crypts.

have negative EMA results, negative tTG results, or both. In many instances, the confusion and problems caused by AGA testing may outweigh the contribution it makes to the correct diagnosis.

43. What is HLA testing?

Sometimes diagnosis of CD may be unclear or confusing. For example, the patient might have a family history of CD, a positive AGA result, and a nonspecific inflammation on small bowel biopsy. If CD cannot be excluded, then **human leucocyte antigen (HLA) testing** may be able to help confirm or rule out the diagnosis. Tests for HLA are genetic tests that determine whether a patient carries a particular gene that predisposes them to a certain trait or disease.

Humans inherit one set of **genes** from each parent and thus carry two sets of genes. Genes control virtually everything in the body. The obvious examples are eye and hair color, your blood type, and height. In addition, genes affect diseases such as cancer, in which the genes that control tissue growth become abnormal, allowing for the unregulated spread and growth of a particular type of cell. This genetic component explains why some diseases tend to run in families: The gene associated with the disease can be passed from parent to child. A gene involved in disease can be present in aunts, uncles, cousins, and grandparents and, if present, can put any family member at risk of developing the disease.

Two genes are associated with CD: HLA-DQ2 and HLA-DQ8. Almost all patients with CD carry one of these genes. Of all patients with CD, about 95 percent have the HLA-DQ2 gene and 5 percent have the HLA-DQ8 gene. Although some other HLA types are associated with CD, the presence of HLA-DQ2 or DQ-8 can be a tool in CD diagnosis.

Approximately 25 to 35 percent of the U.S. population carries HLA-DQ2 or HLA-DQ8, so the presence of the gene is

Human leucocyte antigen (HLA) testing

A blood test to see whether a person carries a specific gene.

Gene

The groups of DNA that are passed from parent to child that determine various body characteristics like eye and hair color.

Evaluation and Diagnosis

not definitive proof of CD because it is so common. Indeed, a positive test for HLA-DQ2 or HLA-DQ8 rarely means the person has CD. However, if the results of blood testing for CD are unclear and the diagnosis cannot be eliminated, negative HLA-DQ2 and/or HLA-DQ8 tests rule out the diagnosis of CD.

HLA testing can be used as an adjunct in testing for CD, but should really be reserved for use by specialists, who have the appropriate resources to deal with the results. Genetic testing can have severe implications for an individual or family, so a genetic counselor should always be made available to anyone who undergoes such tests.

44. What is the "gold standard" when making a diagnosis of celiac disease?

There are many ways to diagnose CD. The last several questions have addressed some of the blood tests for CD, as well as their benefits and limitations. Blood testing can be used to support the diagnosis of CD but does not really produce a definitive answer. The "gold standard" test for CD is the small intestinal biopsy obtained during an endoscopy.

During the endoscopy, the first part of the small intestine is examined visually and the physician has an opportunity to take biopsies (tissue samples). Upon examination, the duodenum can have a normal appearance, be mildly irritated, or demonstrate changes consistent with CD. Duodenal changes seen in CD may include atrophy of the lining of the duodenum, flattening or loss of the normal fold pattern, scalloping of the folds, or a mosaic-appearing mucosa. Identifying these changes on endoscopy is not sufficient for diagnosis, however; rather, a biopsy must be done to confirm the presence of CD. I have seen many normal-appearing duodenums on endoscopy only to have the biopsies reveal the presence of CD. Please see endoscopic examples of a normal and celiac duodenum in Color Plates 1 and 2.

If the results of blood testing for CD are unclear and the diagnosis cannot be eliminated, negative HLA-DQ2 and/or HLA-DQ8 tests rule out the diagnosis of CD.

The "gold standard" test for CD is the small intestinal biopsy obtained during an endoscopy.

The biopsies are mounted on glass slides and processed with various chemicals and stains to help highlight different cells in the specimen. After processing, the slides are examined under the microscope by a specially trained doctor called a pathologist. Normally, the tissue sample will include finger-like projections from the small bowel called villi. A spectrum of damage and inflammation of the villi can be seen by the pathologist and used to diagnose CD, ranging from mild inflammation of the villi to complete loss of the villi. Unfortunately, several other conditions may cause pathologic changes that resemble the damage produced by CD; for example, the changes brought about by severe gastroenteritis or a stomach virus may mimic CD-related changes. Sometimes the biopsy slides need to be sent to an expert pathologist who specializes in diseases of the intestine for a second opinion. In my practice, whenever I see a patient who has been referred by another gastroenterologist, I always request that the slides be sent to me for review by my own pathologists.

It is very important that the biopsies be taken correctly. Patients must be on a gluten-containing diet for at least four weeks prior to taking biopsies. Frequently, patients have a CD screening test by their doctors and are told to start a gluten-free diet and then come in for the endoscopy. As a result of the dietary treatment, the inflammatory changes in the duodenal lining may improve or even completely resolve. As a consequence, beginning a gluten-free diet before endoscopy may result in a false-negative result.

It is recommended that the doctor take at least eight biopsies during the endoscopy to ensure an adequate sample for later analysis. Some centers that specialize in CD employ a technique called "orienting the biopsy." Usually when biopsies are taken they are placed into a jar of formalin, where they float around; the formalin preserves the tissue. In testing for CD, the biopsies should be placed or pinned to a piece of paper so that the villi face up; only then is the tissue placed into the

Patients must be on a gluten-containing diet for at least four weeks prior to taking biopsies. If patients start a gluten-free diet before the endoscopy, the inflammatory changes in the duodenal lining may improve or even completely resolve, leading to a false-negative result.

formalin. Orienting the biopsy allows the pathologist to best visualize the villi.

45. What is endoscopy?

Ambulatory endoscopy center

A free-standing medical procedure center where endoscopy and colonoscopy are done.

An endoscopy test is usually done at a hospital or an **ambulatory endoscopy center,** which is a freestanding facility not associated with a hospital. Generally, a gastroenterologist performs endoscopy, but in some parts of the United States general surgeons, general practitioners, or other physicians may carry out these procedures.

An endoscope is a long, thin instrument that includes a light and a video camera that can be turned in all directions. Air and water can be passed into the endoscope and sucked out, allowing for cleaning retained material or mucus. A variety of tools can be passed down the endoscope—forceps for tissue sampling, cautery probes for treatment of bleeding, and balloons for dilation of the esophagus, to name a few. Video or still pictures can be taken with most endoscopes.

Mucosa

The lining of the intestine.

Clopidogrel (Plavix)

A drug used to thin the blood, thereby preventing heart attack and stroke.

The endoscopy test evaluates the esophagus, stomach, and duodenum (the first part of the small intestine). During the exam, small samples are taken from the lining of the small intestine (the **mucosa**). These biopsies are first processed and then examined under the microscope by a specially trained doctor called a pathologist. They may reveal inflammation and flattening or atrophy of the small intestine villi, suggesting CD.

Warfarin (Coumadin)

A drug used to thin the blood, thereby preventing blood clots.

Do not make any medication changes on your own—ask your doctor.

Prior to undergoing an endoscopy, you will be asked not to eat or drink anything after midnight the night before the test so that your stomach will be empty. The doctor may request minor changes in your medication—for example, not taking blood thinners such as **clopidogrel (Plavix), warfarin (Coumadin),** or aspirin for a few days prior to the examination. Also, diabetic patients must change their insulin dosing. Do not make any medication changes on your own—ask your doctor. Also, do not go to an endoscopy test alone. You will likely be sedated and given medication for relaxation or sleep during the procedure, so you will not be able to drive after the test. Someone will need to drive you home.

Overall, the time from your arrival at the center to your departure will be about 2 hours. Of that time, the actual exam takes only 10 to 15 minutes. A nurse or doctor will do an interview, asking about your medical history, any medications that you are taking, your symptoms, and any drug allergies. A limited physical exam is then done to ensure that anesthesia or sedation can be administered to you safely. An **intravenous (IV) line** will be placed so that the sedative medication can be given.

Next, you will be brought into the procedure room. Monitors for your oxygen level, heart rhythm and rate, and blood pressure will be placed on your arms and chest. Everyone gets supplemental oxygen because some people do not breathe well while sedated. All of this occurs prior to starting the actual endoscopy test.

Once all of the preparation is complete, a nurse or anesthesiologist will administer the sedative. Patients may sleep through the exam and not remember it, or they may simply be sleepy throughout the procedure—it depends on the doctor and medications used for sedation. The mouth is usually sprayed or you may gargle with a topical anesthetic to numb the throat so that the instrument can be easily passed through it. The topical anesthetic also helps to prevent you from gagging and is generally very effective even with patients who gag easily.

Once you are sedated, an endoscope is passed into your mouth down the esophagus, into the stomach, and then into the duodenum, where the biopsies are taken. Testing for CD always includes a biopsy of the small intestine that is taken during endoscopy for later examination under the microscope. Celiac

Evaluation and Diagnosis

Intravenous (IV) line

The placement of a needle in the patient's blood vessel, which is then used to infuse fluid into the patient's bloodstream.

Testing for CD always includes a biopsy of the small intestine that is taken during endoscopy for later examination under the microscope. Celiac disease is not a visual diagnosis, so the visual inspection may reveal abnormalities, or the tissue may look normal despite microscopic changes.

disease is not a visual diagnosis, so the visual inspection may reveal abnormalities, or the tissue may look normal despite microscopic changes.

After the exam, patients are brought to a recovery room and sleep off the sedative, which may take 30 to 60 minutes. This is really the only "recovery" from the exam necessary, because no cuts or incisions are made and the test does not lead to any pain. Most doctors recommend that you not drive, work, exercise, consume alcohol, or make important decisions on the day of the exam because it takes about 24 hours for the sedative medication to completely clear from your system. It is important that you avoid alcohol for 24 hours because it can interact with any medication that remains in your system.

46. Is endoscopy painful, and does it carry risks?

Endoscopy is a safe and routine procedure. The major risks relate to the anesthesia.

Endoscopy is a safe and routine procedure. The major risks relate to the anesthesia administered during the exam. On rare occasions, patients may have allergic reactions to the medications. The anesthetic risks are generally cardiac (heart related) and pulmonary (lung related). Examples include irregular heart rates or, very rarely, heart attack. These complications may occur in patients with a history of heart disease or lung disease.

The major risk during the actual endoscopy exam is bleeding or perforation. A perforation is a tear in the lining of the esophagus or stomach. On rare occasions, it may require a hospital stay, blood transfusion, or surgery to fix the tear. All of these risks or complications are exceedingly rare, occurring in fewer than 1 in 1000 procedures.

Overall, endoscopy is not painful—no cutting or incisions are made. The placement of an IV hurts but is quick. Sometimes the initial passage of the scope through the throat into the

esophagus is a little uncomfortable because it is an unusual feeling to swallow the endoscope. The most common issue patients experience is a sore throat that lasts for a couple of days after the procedure; the soreness occurs because the scope travels through the back of the throat and can cause some irritation. The other issue may be some dizziness or nausea after the endoscopy related to the sedative medication—its side effects sometimes include nausea. This problem is easily treated and usually short-lived. I have had an endoscopy, and I do not remember a thing about it and did not find it to be an unpleasant experience.

One issue patients often ask about is the risk of infection—that is, the chance of catching something from the exam. Such problems are very rare because endoscopes are cleaned carefully, with sterilizing solutions being pumped through the instrument between each examination. Yes, endoscopes are reused many times, but their cleaning is standardized and regulated by the federal agencies that license hospitals and freestanding endoscopy units or surgical centers.

Before your endoscopy procedure, the nurse or preferably the doctor will review all of the risks and the benefits of the examination with you. This conversation offers an opportunity for you to discuss the actual procedure and to learn what the doctor is going to do and why. Any unresolved questions or issues that you have should be addressed at this meeting. You will then sign an **informed consent** form. The informed consent restates the risks of the exam. By signing it, you acknowledge that you understand the risks and agree to go ahead with the procedure.

47. Why do I need a biopsy of the small intestine, and does it hurt?

The purpose of doing the endoscopy is to obtain biopsies of the duodenum, which can then be examined by a pathologist

Informed consent
A form signed by the patient or his or her medical proxy that acknowledges the risks and benefits associated with a medical procedure.

for microscopic changes of inflammation. Biopsies should be done regardless of what the duodenum looks like during endoscopy. Frequently, the endoscopy looks completely normal. In such cases, patients may become frustrated, asking why they needed the exam, only to have the biopsy show CD a few days later. Changes seen on endoscopy can range from normal to mild irritation or redness to flattening of the normal folds and **scalloping of the mucosa**. Because of these issues, biopsies are completely mandatory, as you want to make completely sure the diagnosis is correct before going on a gluten-free diet for life.

Scalloping of the mucosa

An abnormality seen on endoscopic examination of the duodenum; it requires biopsy to confirm celiac disease.

Biopsies are mandatory, as you want to make completely sure the diagnosis is correct before going on a gluten-free diet for life.

Taking biopsies is very safe. During the endoscopy, several tiny pinches of tissue are removed through the scope. It is generally suggested to take about eight biopsies, as this number improves the chances of detecting the appropriate tissue changes. The biopsies add about five minutes to the endoscopic exam. On very rare occasions, the patient may experience bleeding from biopsy site, develop an infection, or have a hole poked through the lining of the duodenum. I have never seen any of these complications in my career and I feel that this risk is negligible.

The nerves of the gut do not feel pinching, cutting, or burning, so the biopsies are painless. These nerves do feel stretching, pulling, and distention from the scope or air that is used during the procedure, which results in stomach cramps that last only a few minutes. I tell my patients that if they are willing to have an endoscopy, then biopsies are part of the package.

Marye comments:

I did not find the endoscopy painful, nor did I have any after effects from it. The most difficult part of the test for me was finding a vein from which to obtain blood for testing.

48. What do the small intestine and villi normally do?

The gut (gastrointestinal tract or intestines) is a hollow, muscular tube that spans from the mouth to the anus. Although its length varies from person to person, it generally spans 20 to 25 feet. The major job of the GI tract is the processing and digestion of food and nutrients and the storage and elimination of waste. The pancreas and the liver aid in this process by producing bile and digestive enzymes that break down food products into absorbable nutrients. Each part of the GI tract has a special function in food processing. (See Figure 3.)

The mouth and teeth provide mechanical chewing of food to break large pieces down into smaller pieces. Oral saliva lubricates this mass of food and contains enzymes that start the digestion of complex sugars. The esophagus is a muscular tube that moves food from the mouth to the stomach.

The stomach serves as a reservoir for food. This strong muscle pumps food and liquid around like a washing machine, bathing food in acid and breaking it down further into increasingly smaller particles. In addition, the stomach has other jobs, such as making digestive enzymes and acid, and helping with the digestion of vitamins such as vitamin B_{12}. The stomach also works as a gatekeeper, slowly letting liquefied acidic food trickle into the small intestine.

The small intestine is made up of three parts: the duodenum, the jejunum, and the ileum. Celiac disease may affect all three of these components. During the endoscopy, the duodenum is biopsied predominantly because that is as far down as most standard endoscopes go (some scopes go farther but are generally used only on special occasions). In the duodenum, liquefied nutrients mix with bile from the liver and enzymes from the pancreas. Owing to their actions, the small intestine is the major site of digestion—that is, breaking down large pieces of food into simple proteins, fats, and sugars that are suitable for absorption. The small intestine is 12 to 20 feet long and features a series of folds; it is lined with microscopic finger-like projections called villi (Figure 6).

The villi are where digested food material is absorbed into the bloodstream. As part of the digestion process, they make enzymes that break down sugars and protein. For example, the villi manufacture lactase (the enzyme that is lost in lactose intolerance). When CD is present, the villi become inflamed and do not make enzymes or absorb digested nutrients properly. The reason the small intestine is so long and contains so many villi is to maximize the surface area of the gut that is exposed to digested food. If you could spread the small bowel and villi out in full, they would cover an entire tennis court!

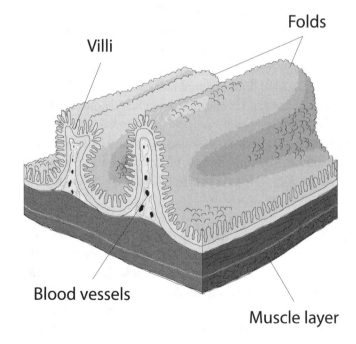

Small Intestine Lining

Figure 6   Cartoon cross section of the duodenum, showing a normal fold with the overlaying mucosa that contains the villi.

In addition to digesting and absorbing nutrients from food, the small intestine acts as a pump, moving liquid from the stomach downstream to the colon. In CD, this pumping action is weak or abnormal. As a consequence, things slow down, giving bacteria more opportunities to grow. The resulting bacterial overgrowth further impairs digestion and absorption.

Each part of the small intestine has a different function, and certain nutrients are absorbed at particular sites. For example, the duodenum and first part of the jejunum absorb dietary iron, which is used to produce red blood cells. These areas are affected in CD, a phenomenon that explains why anemia is one of the most common manifestations of CD. Of course, CD can also involve the entire small intestine, resulting in abnormal absorption of other vitamins, protein, and fat and leading to diarrhea and weight loss. The last part of the small intestine, called the ileum, normally absorbs vitamin B_{12} and bile salts. If CD involves the ileum, a vitamin B_{12} deficiency and bile salt malabsorption can occur, resulting in anemia and diarrhea.

The last part of the gut is the colon (large intestine), which has two major functions: absorption of fluid and storage. The colon takes up about a liter of fluid, making the stool solid. The storage function allows for control of a bowel movement until facilities are available. There are no villi in the colon, and for the most part the colon does not really absorb nutrients. Usually, the colon is not involved in CD, although an inflammatory condition of the colon called microscopic colitis can complicate CD.

49. What changes are seen in the biopsy of celiac disease? What is the Marsh level?

Historically, CD has been associated with damage and inflammation of the small intestine. The severity of this damage can run the gamut from mild irritation associated with specialized inflammatory cells (called lymphocytes) present in the villi to complete destruction of the villi (atrophy). These abnormalities were first described and categorized by a pathologist named Marsh. Today, the various degrees of changes on small intestine biopsy that correlate to the amount of damage or symptoms from CD are identified in standardized terms known as the **Marsh levels**. Thus, when a pathologist examines a biopsy under the microscope, he or she can assign a Marsh level, which pathologists all over the world would understand as a means of grading abnormalities (also known as "staging the disease").

Marsh levels

The system used to grade the inflammation seen under the microscope in biopsies with celiac disease.

Part of the Marsh grading system focuses on atrophy of the villi (Figure 7). When viewed under a microscope, the villi resemble a shag rug. With increasing inflammation and damage, they atrophy (become shorter and shorter) until the villi completely disappear. Please see Color Plates 3 and 4, color microscopic photos of normal duodenum and villi (CP3), and the same from a patient with CD (CP4). The higher the Marsh level, the more severe the symptoms and more likely that the antibody test for CD will be positive.

Although flattening and atrophy of the villi are seen in CD, these changes can also occur with some other diseases. Severe

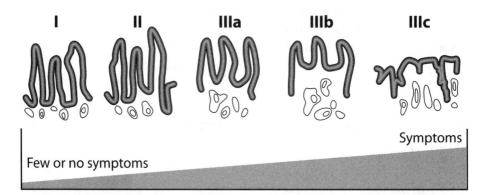

Figure 7 Marsh staging is used to classify progressive damage to villi caused by celiac disease. The stages range from stage I (normal) to stage IIIc (complete flattening of the villi). (From AGA technical review on celiac disease. Gastro 2006 Rostum, Murray, Kagnoff)

gastroenteritis (stomach flu), for example, may cause similar changes on small intestine biopsy. Likewise, bacterial overgrowth of the small intestine causes inflammation of the villi. Biopsies in cases involving tropical sprue can look exactly the same as those taken from patients with CD; antibody testing will be negative in patients with tropical sprue, however, and the appropriate history with a visit to the tropics is required to distinguish the tropical disease. As mentioned, the small intestine biopsy is mandatory for diagnosis of CD, but it needs to be done in the correct scenario. Positive blood testing, a family history of CD, or a picture of malabsorption are all supportive of CD, and the appropriate biopsy confirms the diagnosis.

Biopsies are examined under the microscope by a pathologist. Their interpretation is subjective, meaning the pathologist gives an opinion based on his or her experience and training. This is not a black-and-white process, but rather involves shades of gray. For instance, pathologists at smaller community hospitals may not see many small bowel biopsies or cases of CD. For these reasons, it might be reasonable to "get a second opinion" and have the biopsies reviewed elsewhere. In my practice, when I see a patient who has been referred with possible CD, I request his or her biopsies for review by a specially trained gastrointestinal pathologist. On rare occasions, if there is a lingering question about the interpretation of the biopsies, I might send them out for review by expert pathologists.

50. What is a capsule endoscopy?

Physicians use a variety of diagnostic procedures to identify the presence of CD. Imaging the small intestine is difficult because of its length—12 to 20 feet—and its many twists and turns, which make doing an endoscopic exam of the entire small intestine nearly impossible. Several types of very long scopes can be used for this purpose; however, these tests may be limited in availability and require travel to a large referral hospital or teaching hospital. Small bowel endoscopy generally takes a long time because of the length of the structure that needs to be examined, and it requires sedation because the test is uncomfortable. Nevertheless, when used appropriately in selected patients, these procedures are very useful tests.

Direct visual examination of the small bowel was originally developed for patients with chronic gastrointestinal bleeding with an obscure source. Careful examination of the small intestine was found to be able to show ulcers, abnormal blood vessels, and bleeding lesions. With further use and wider indications, other abnormalities were found with such examinations, such as Crohn's disease, tumors, and CD. The value offered by such tests has led to many new uses for small bowel endoscopy.

Because of the limitations of direct visual examination of the small intestine, the market was open for an easier and painless alternative for examining this organ. Capsule endoscopy, also known as the "PillCam," is one such option. In this case, the **capsule endoscope** is a pill the size of a large vitamin that contains a light source, a color video camera, and a transmitter (Figure 8).

Capsule endoscope

A pill that is an endoscope.

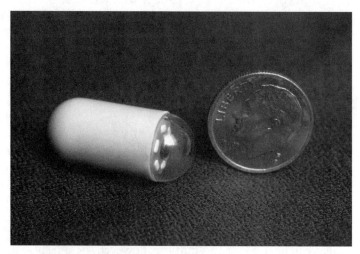

Figure 8   The capsule endoscope.

In capsule endoscopy, the patient wears several electrical leads that are taped or stuck onto the abdomen. The leads are connected to a receiver/recording device that is worn on a belt. There are no needles, and the test is painless. To perform the test, the patient fasts for a brief period of time (usually 10 hours), goes to the doctor's office, and then swallows the capsule. The patient is then free to leave and perform his or her usual activities. The capsule travels down the esophagus, into the stomach, and through the entire small intestine. During its travels through the gut, the camera takes video pictures many times a minute and transmits the images to the recording belt. The duration of the test is limited by the battery life of the capsule (eight hours), although this amount of time is generally adequate to examine most, if not all, of the small intestine. Ultimately, the capsule is passed in a normal bowel movement and the pill is "flushed" away.

When the exam is finished (on the same day the patient swallows the capsule), the patient returns to the doctor's office, and the electrical leads and recording belt are removed. The information in the recorder is downloaded to a computer. Using special software, the doctor is able to view all of the images obtained over the eight-hour period. The doctor can tell roughly where the pill is in the intestine when a particular image is reviewed. Images can be saved on CDs, and pictures of abnormalities can be printed.

Capsule endoscopy does have some limitations. Many insurance carriers will not pay for a capsule exam, and I recommend that payment issues be resolved with your doctor's office prior to the exam to avoid a large bill (some exams cost more than $1000). Occasionally, the pill stays in the stomach and does not travel into the small intestine during the eight-hour life of the battery. In such a case, the exam would be inadequate and on rare occasions the doctor may have to do an endoscopy test to place another capsule into the small intestine.

The major medical risk associated with the capsule exam is the pill getting stuck somewhere and causing a **bowel obstruction**. Patients who have had prior intestinal surgery, prior bowel obstructions, and strictures of the small intestine such as those in Crohn's disease are at increased risk for this complication. If the capsule does cause a bowel obstruction, surgery will be required to remove the capsule, though this happens very rarely.

The capsule cannot take a biopsy, which is its greatest limitation in terms of diagnosing CD (biopsies are mandatory for CD diagnosis). Thus capsule endoscopy probably will never play a major role in the initial diagnosis of CD. Instead, it is a diagnostic tool that can be helpful in certain situations, such as determining the source of chronic obscure GI bleeding and looking for a bleeding site that might occur in CD. In my practice, I have found the capsule helpful in diagnosing complications of CD such as ulcerative jejunitis and lymphoma and for investigating an abnormality on a barium x-ray of the small intestine. The capsule study can also provide valuable information in those CD patients with ongoing unexplained weight loss. Capsule endoscopy is widely available throughout the world because of its ease of performance.

51. What is a barium study?

The condition of CD with weight loss and diarrhea and its relationship to wheat proteins have been recognized for decades. Celiac disease involves the small intestine—historically, this is a very difficult area to examine or get tissue samples. **Barium studies** (also known as **upper GI series** or **small bowel follow-through**) were one of the earliest tools used to make this diagnosis; they have been performed for more than 100 years. Barium is a thick liquid that you drink during the exam, after which multiple x-rays are taken (Figure 9). The barium coats the lining of the gut, and its imaging can give great information about the esophagus, stomach, and small intestine, including the classic findings in CD. These x-ray exams remain a helpful tool in the diagnosis and ongoing management of CD. Studies can be followed over time to see whether any changes have occurred. Complications of CD such as **ulcerative jejunitis** and **intestinal lymphoma**, for example, are easily diagnosed with barium.

Barium studies are generally performed at your local hospital and require a doctor's orders. The exam is fairly painless and includes an intravenous (IV) line, which will cause discomfort; in addition, sometimes the barium can cause cramps. After the IV is placed, several glasses of barium are swallowed while x-rays are taken. The examination of the small intestine—the key component of this test—usually takes about 2 hours (though the actual time can be quite variable). As the barium passes through your intestines, the technician or doctor may press on your abdomen with a device that looks like a large spoon to move things around.

Ulcerative jejunitis

A refractory type of celiac disease that can evolve into lymphoma.

Intestinal lymphoma

A cancer of the lymph nodes involving the small intestine. Also known as enteropathy-associated T-cell lymphoma.

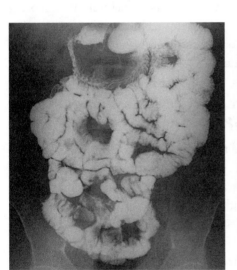
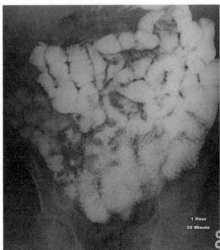

Figure 9 An x-ray examination of the small intestine in which barium (the white material) is used to coat the lining of the intestine. Normal exam is on the left. The right example is from a patient with CD; the x-ray demonstrates abnormal-appearing folds and dilution or thinning of the barium.

Evaluation and Diagnosis

Patients voice some concerns about radiation exposure. In reality, the amount of radiation to which you are subjected during an x-ray examination is relatively small. When you are flying in an airplane, you are exposed to cosmic radiation; your radiation exposure during an upper GI exam is roughly equal to that of two roundtrip flights from New York to Los Angeles. This small amount of radiation should not be of concern, although I would not recommend having regular or annual x-rays.

Once developed, the x-rays are read by a radiologist, a doctor who specializes in their interpretation. Abnormalities of the gut lining may include irritation, ulcers, scarring, strictures (narrowing), and cancer. Barium examination can diagnose any of these conditions involving the esophagus, stomach, and small intestine. For this reason, barium studies are still done regularly despite the availability of more modern tools such as computed tomography (CT) scans and magnetic resonance imaging (MRI), which may not be as helpful in diagnosing CD. The major drawback of this technique when diagnosing CD (besides the minor discomfort) is that tissue sampling or biopsies cannot be done.

52. Which other tests can be used for diagnosis of celiac disease?

The major tools used to diagnose CD are the three blood tests discussed in detail in Question 38: the antiendomysial antibody, tissue transglutaminase antibody, and (rarely) the antigliadin antibody. Endoscopy and biopsy of the small intestine will confirm the diagnosis if the appropriate inflammatory changes are found. If the diagnosis is in doubt or the picture is unclear, then a barium study or small bowel x-ray may be helpful in ruling CD in or out. Likewise, a capsule endoscopy may play a role in confirming or excluding the diagnosis.

Frequently, patients with CD have diarrhea, so stool studies checking for an infection or parasites are mandatory. For those individuals with diarrhea, sometimes a 72-hour stool collection might be done. During this test, the patient eats a high-fat diet; the stool is then collected over a three-day period. This study helps to quantify how much diarrhea is occurring and identify whether the patient is absorbing fat normally or if the fat is passing undigested into the stool, thereby causing diarrhea.

Most patients with diarrhea should undergo a colonoscopy with biopsy of the lining of the colon. Colonoscopy usually is a colon cancer screening test that, in younger persons, is reserved for those with a family history of colon cancer or polyps; it is recommended at age 50 as a more general screening measure for colon cancer. Nevertheless, such an examination is also very helpful for evaluation of patients with chronic diarrhea.

A colonoscopy is very similar to an endoscopy. Prior to the exam, you must eat a limited diet for a few days, avoiding roughage. The day before the test, you drink a laxative solution to clean out your bowels. You will need a ride to and from the test, as you will be sedated and possibly put to sleep with medication during the actual procedure and cannot drive afterward.

The actual exam takes about 30 minutes. It begins with a rectal examination. The colonoscope is then placed into the rectum and moved throughout the entire colon, possibly going as far as the last part of the small intestine. This technique allows for direct visual examination of the lining of the colon, removal of any polyps (which can be precancerous), and the ability to take biopsies.

All patients with chronic diarrhea need to have biopsies done, as the colonoscopy may show only normal tissue, only to have the biopsy reveal an abnormal inflammation called microscopic colitis. Question 24 discusses microscopic colitis and its relationship to CD.

Blood testing in addition to CD-specific tests should be done to check for anemia, and a thyroid test should be performed as well when CD is suspected. An overactive thyroid (hyperthyroidism) manifests as diarrhea and weight loss and so can mimic CD. Individuals with CD should have their liver tests checked, as these tests can be a clue to nutritional status and may help diagnose any associated liver diseases. Other blood tests, such as those for inflammation, kidney tests, and vitamin levels, can also be helpful.

Many patients ask whether they need a CT or MRI scan. For any patient with unexplained weight loss, a CT scan of the abdomen and pelvis should be done just to ensure that no masses or cancer is present. This is usually adequate in the case of CD. I am not a big fan of performing MRI scans unless the doctor knows exactly what he or she is looking for. One new MRI test does scan the small intestine much like a barium x-ray and could potentially provide valuable information in those patients who experience ongoing weight loss despite following a strict gluten-free diet. At the moment, it is not widely available.

53. Which other evaluations should be done when a patient is newly diagnosed with celiac disease?

Once a diagnosis of CD is made, further testing is needed to check for other diseases that can be present or that can complicate CD. Some of these tests may have been done in the evaluation of weight loss or diarrhea. Blood work recommended comprises a complete blood count to check for anemia, liver tests, thyroid tests, and some vitamin levels. In my practice, I test my patients' folic acid, vitamin B_{12}, and vitamin D levels; I also test three mineral levels—calcium, iron, and zinc. These vitamins and minerals are poorly absorbed when a person has CD so their levels may be low, requiring supplementation. You should discuss the specific tests recommended for you with your doctor.

Patients with CD do not absorb dietary fat normally, which means that their absorption of certain vitamins that are taken up with fat (called fat-soluble vitamins) is affected by their disease. Vitamin D, a fat-soluble vitamin responsible for healthy bones, is frequently low in CD, increasing risk of the patient's osteoporosis (thinning of the bones). Other risk factors for osteoporosis include female sex, living in a cold climate with insufficient sun exposure, Caucasian race, being thin, smoking, lack of exercise, and family history of osteoporosis. Dairy products such as yogurt, milk, and cheese are excellent sources of vitamin D. Vitamin D is also made by the skin when it is exposed to the sun; thus not getting regular sun exposure can result in vitamin D deficiency. In my practice, I always check the calcium and vitamin D levels in patients who are newly diagnosed with CD and supplement them as needed. More generally, it is recommended that women take 1200 mg of calcium and 800 units of vitamin D per day to prevent osteoporosis, regardless of whether they have CD. This supplementation is even more important in CD.

All patients newly diagnosed with CD should also undergo a bone density scan. This painless exam uses low-level x-rays to measure how dense the bones are. It can tell whether the bones are of normal density, mildly thinned (osteopenia), or very thin (osteoporosis). The bone density scan can be repeated every year or two to follow bone health. If osteoporosis is diagnosed, a variety of medications are available for treatment. This issue is very important because osteoporosis increases a person's risk of experiencing bone fractures as he or she ages. When an affected individual has osteoporosis, fractures can occur even with minor trauma, such as stubbing a toe and breaking it. More seriously, an individual might fall and break a hip, which requires surgery to repair the damage. Some fractures may arise spontaneously, in the absence of trauma. For example, a vertebral compression fracture occurs when one of the bones (vertebrae) in the spine collapses, resulting in loss of height, pain, and bending or twisting of the spine.

Evaluation and Diagnosis

Other vitamin levels may be ordered depending on your particular symptoms. For example, your vitamin A levels might be checked. **Vitamin A** is a fat-soluble vitamin that promotes healthy vision; low levels of this vitamin may produce night blindness (difficulty seeing at night). If a blood vitamin A level or **carotene** level confirms such a deficiency, the patient should begin supplementation with beta carotene. In my practice, I usually recommend that all patients with CD take a gluten-free multivitamin to avoid some of these issues.

Vitamin A

A fat-soluble vitamin required for vision and skin health.

Carotene

A form of vitamin A that aids healthy vision.

Table 13   Recommended Testing after a New Diagnosis of Celiac Disease

Test	Reason
Complete blood count (CBC)	Test for anemia
Liver function tests (LFTs)	Test for nutrition and liver disease
Thyroid test (TSH)	Tests thyroid function
Iron, transferring and ferritin	Test for iron status
Calcium level	Test for bones
Vitamin D level	Test for bones
Folic acid/Folate	Test for anemia
Vitamin B$_{12}$ level	Tests for anemia and nerve function
Carotene (vitamin A test)	Vitamin responsible for vision
Bone density scan	Test for bone health and osteoporosis

PART FIVE

Treatment for Celiac Disease: The Gluten-Free Diet

What is gluten?

What is a gluten-free diet?

Should I see a dietitian?

More . . .

54. What is gluten?

Gluten is a protein found in wheat and similar grains (such as rye and barley). It gives wheat dough an elastic or sticky property, allowing it to be kneaded and stretched. Gluten proteins are not well digested and remain partially intact as they pass through the stomach and into the small intestine. One gluten protein, called gliadin, is particularly resistant to digestion. Gliadin stimulates a very strong response of inflammation, activating the immune system in the celiac small intestine. The immune system reacts to the gliadin protein by creating an antibody to bind this foreign protein when it is present. One of the tests for CD is the antigliadin antibody (AGA), which can be measured in the blood.

The presence of gluten in food can be obvious: The label may plainly state that wheat, rye, or barley is an ingredient, as in breads or pasta. Other foodstuffs and cooking agents may contain gluten proteins but not make their presence obvious or even note them on the label. *You must read all the labels of all the foods you consume to avoid inadvertently ingesting gluten.* Gluten-containing ingredients to look for on labels include malt products, **barley malt extract,** hydrolyzed wheat protein, hydrolyzed vegetable or plant protein, teriyaki, soy sauce, modified food starch, brown rice syrup, dextrin, and vegetable gum. If you are not sure, then do not eat the foodstuff.

Gluten protein, which is inexpensive, is often added to food because of its sticky glue-like properties. This property also makes gluten attractive for use in other products—for example, cosmetics, medications, and even stationery products. Gluten is frequently added to prescription and over-the-counter medications as a filler or binder, though it may not be listed on the drug label. You should ask your pharmacist whether a specific medication is gluten-free; if any question remains, contact the drug manufacturer directly for more information.

Gluten-containing ingredients to look for on labels include malt products, barley malt extract, hydrolyzed wheat protein, hydrolyzed vegetable or plant protein, teriyaki, soy sauce, modified food starch, brown rice syrup, dextrin, and vegetable gum.

Barley extract (barley malt)

A gluten-containing food additive.

Lists of gluten-free medications can also be downloaded from the Internet. For instance, several downloadable lists of gluten-free drugs from a celiac conference sponsored by the Northeastern Ohio University College of Medicine can be found at www.glutenfreedrugs.com/. Another excellent (and downloadable) list of safe medications is available from the Wheaton Gluten-free support group at http://homepage.mac.com/sholland/celiac/GFmedlist.pdf.

Marye comments:

Gluten is a protein found in many foods, such as pasta, bread, cereal, vitamins, prescriptions, soy sauce, tomato soup, creams, sauces, gravies, some cold cuts, toothpaste, lipstick, envelopes, and so many other things. It is important to read labels prior to eating or buying the item.

55. Which grains must be avoided in celiac disease?

Gluten-containing grains include wheat, rye, barley, and possibly oats. Confusing matters further is the fact that there are many different types and species of these grains, which go by many different names (see Table 14). These grains and the products derived from them are toxic to patients with CD and must be removed from the diet. The issue of oats is discussed separately in Question 61, as there is some debate about whether oats are safe to eat if you have CD. Nevertheless, because of the possibility of contamination with gluten, you should avoid most oat preparations when you are on a gluten-free diet.

Any foods or products made with any of these grains must be avoided, because they can contain gluten. For this reason, you should always read food labels carefully, searching for any potentially questionable ingredients or additives.

Table 14   Toxic Grains to Be Avoided in Celiac Disease

Barley	Kamut
Barley malt	Matzo flour/meal
Barley extract	Orzo
Bulgur	Panko
Couscous	Rye
Dinkle	Seitan
Durum	Semolina
Einkorn	Spelt
Emmer	Triticale
Farina	Udon
Faro?	Wheat bran, germ, or starch
Graham flour	Oats?

Marye comments:

I have found it is best to avoid all grains except corn or rice that has been processed on machinery that has not processed any other grains, so that contamination has not taken place.

56. What is a gluten-free diet?

A gluten-free diet is a diet prescribed by a doctor for patients who have an allergy to gluten proteins. It is required for patients with CD and dermatitis herpetiformis. Some patients may have gastrointestinal symptoms and not have a true allergy but rather a sensitivity to gluten. Although these individuals do not have CD, they may still benefit from following a gluten-free or gluten-restricted diet.

A true gluten-free diet is completely free of any source of gluten proteins. High vigilance is required to avoid gluten in the form of known or unknown food ingredients, flavorings, cross-contamination of food, or nonfood exposures. Knowledge of toxic grains and food additives that may contain gluten is key to achieving this goal. Reading lists of ingredients and scrutinizing food labels are mandatory if you want to comply with the diet. In particular, you must be aware of potential sources of gluten other than the conventional items such as bread or pasta. These sources can include medications, cosmetics, the glue on envelopes and stamps, and religious items such as communion wafers. All food ingredients must be examined for the buzzwords that may signify contamination, such as "malt," "dextrin," or "hydrolyzed plant proteins."

Some food labels state they are gluten-free. Unfortunately, "gluten-free" may be a relative term, because the United States does not currently have any regulation that governs gluten labeling, and a variety of definitions of this term exist. The Gluten Intolerance Group deems foods to be safe if they contain fewer than 10 parts gluten per million parts product. In Canada and some other countries, "gluten-free" is defined as no obvious added gluten and fewer than 20 parts gluten per million parts product. Sensitivity to gluten varies among celiac patients, and some may become symptomatic even when they ingest even these small amounts. Establishment of a U.S. federal standard related to gluten is in the works and may become available within the next two years.

A gluten-free diet is just that—completely free of all gluten. It does not mean following a gluten-free diet during the week with time off on the weekends or having a slice of white bread or beer periodically. The gluten-free diet must be learned. The initial education is provided by from a dietitian, which requires a consultation. Follow-up appointments are then needed to handle any questions and to ensure that the appropriate foods are avoided. The dietitian meeting is just the first part of the journey, however, and many other resources are available and should be utilized to help you along the way.

There are many intricacies to negotiating the gluten-free diet that go beyond the scope of this book and could take up hundreds of pages. Indeed, it would be nearly impossible to cover the entire topic of CD, DH, and gluten-free eating in one book. Even so, you cannot have too much information on the gluten-free diet. Dietitians are highly qualified for this task, given that they routinely work to educate patients on specific dietary issues. An excellent resource regarding the gluten-free diet is the book *Gluten-Free Diet* by Shelley Case, an expert dietitian who writes extensively on CD and diet.

Support groups can be of tremendous help in learning the diet and identifying which foods may be safe. The Celiac Sprue Association (CSA) publishes the *CSA Gluten-Free Guide*, now available in its eleventh edition (www.csaceliacs.org; 1-877-CSA-4-CSA). This organization's motto is "Celiacs helping celiacs," which is exactly what its guide does. The CSA guide is highly recommended and contains a discussion of the gluten-free diet as well as lists of gluten-free food products, cosmetic products, markets, restaurants, medications, religious products, food manufacturers, and even arts-and-crafts supplies.

A brief downloadable review of the gluten-free diet, a list of safe and toxic grains, and a sample shopping list is available from the North American Society of Pediatric Gastroenterology, Hepatology, and Nutrition (NASPGHAN) at www.naspghan.org/assets/diseaseInfo/pdf/GlutenFreeDietGuide-E.pdf. This site is a good place to start what can seem like an overwhelming journey. To complement its information, I strongly suggest that you purchase a more comprehensive gluten-free food guide as well.

A point of debate is the need to follow a gluten-free diet if you have potential or latent CD. These patients have no symptoms, positive blood tests, and normal small bowel biopsies. Other individuals may have had CD as children but "grew out of it." The general recommendation for latent CD is *not* to treat it with a gluten-free diet.

57. Is there a medication or pill I can take to cure my celiac disease?

The short answer to this question is no—the current treatment for CD is a gluten-free diet. There is, however, some promising research in this area. Medication-related studies are investigating several possible avenues to approach the disease, including enzyme preparations to help digest toxic gluten and gliadin proteins, drugs to help decrease gut inflammation, and vaccines.

Dietary gluten and gliadin proteins are resistant to digestion by stomach acid and pancreatic enzymes in humans. As a result, they remain intact on their way to the small intestine, initiating the allergic response. Recently, researchers at Stanford University published a study on combination enzyme therapy using a human model of CD. These scientists created a two-enzyme "cocktail" whose components worked in a complementary fashion, both digesting and inactivating dietary gluten and gliadin. One component of this cocktail is **EP-B2,** an enzyme derived from barley that works under stomach conditions. The other component, **PEP,** is an enzyme derived from bacteria that works under duodenal conditions. In the lab, the enzyme cocktail fully detoxified store-bought gluten in 10 minutes in simulated conditions found in the human duodenum. Immune cells obtained from celiac patients at endoscopy did not react to the treated gluten, nor did antigluten antibodies.

Other studies are investigating the role of enzyme supplements that can digest toxic proteins, thereby blocking the allergic response. In the future, these medications might be used in much the same way as the lactase supplements that are currently available to help people with lactose intolerance.

The gut acts as a barrier to keep some things in the nutrient stream out and allow only certain molecules in. Cells lining the intestines are linked together with so-called **tight junctions**— "gates" that keep small molecules from sneaking in between cells. **Zonulin** is a protein that sends signals to open the tight junction gates, allowing more molecules in. The level of zonulin found in the body is increased in inflammatory conditions of

EP-B2

An enzyme that digests gluten. It is currently being studied as a treatment for celiac disease.

PEP

A type of enzyme being studied as a treatment for celiac disease.

Tight junctions

The protein structures that hold together the cells that line the small intestine.

Zonulin

A protein that helps regulate the movement of nutrients into the cells lining the villi.

AT-1001

An investigational drug not yet approved by the U.S. Food and Drug Administration that is being studied for celiac disease. It blocks zonulin, keeping the gut from becoming leaky in the setting of inflammation.

the gut such as CD and Crohn's disease, resulting in a leaky (that is, more permeable) gut. **AT-1001** is an oral medication under development that blocks the action of zonulin. When this drug was tested in patients with CD who were given a gluten challenge, results were very positive. AT-1001 was well tolerated with no side effects, and symptoms of gluten toxicity were inhibited in the AT-1001 group compared with members of a control group who took a sugar pill (placebo). Laboratory measures of gut permeability also demonstrated that the intestinal barrier function was maintained with administration of AT-1001.

The studies mentioned here focused on the two most promising potential treatments for CD. More research is in progress looking at these and other agents that may eventually allow persons with CD to consume small amounts of gluten. At the same time, a drug to treat CD and allow patients to have a normal diet currently does not exist and is likely many years away. Nevertheless, there is great interest in this area among patients, doctors, scientists, and the pharmaceutical companies that provide the financial backing for these CD-related projects, so an effective treatment remains highly sought after.

58. Should I see a dietitian?

The answer to this question is a resounding yes! The gluten-free diet is a potential minefield. If you inadvertently eat gluten, you may become sick and cause chronic damage to your small intestine, putting you at risk for the complications of CD. A dietitian provides education about the gluten-free diet; follow-up appointments are like a test to see if you understand the concepts explained in previous meetings. The dietitian can help you comply with the diet by recommending gluten-free foods, manufacturers that produce gluten-free products, supermarkets that specialize in celiac-friendly foods, and restaurants that may be safe. He or she can also recommend strategies to help you avoid gluten both at home and when eating at restaurants.

Another major role of the dietitian is to go through your current diet to see if there are any problems with it. Frequently, newly diagnosed patients begin the diet but continue to have symptoms, typically as a result of unknown gluten ingestion. On other occasions, a patient with longstanding CD may suddenly develop symptoms after years of following a strict diet. The dietitian can carefully examine the diet to identify potential problem areas.

Celiac disease causes malabsorption so that food is not completely absorbed, resulting in diarrhea with loss of nutrients and weight. After a few months on the gluten-free diet, this damage to the small intestine heals and food is then absorbed normally. For example, if a patient with untreated CD eats 2000 calories per day, he or she may absorb only 80 to 90 percent of that amount, or about 1700 calories. If the individual then goes on a gluten-free diet and eats the same amount, the intestinal damage will heal and the person will absorb the full 2000 calories. Thus, although the person is eating the same number of calories, he or she is actually taking in 300 more calories per day. This change very commonly results in weight gain—which is good if you are underweight but can lead to obesity if maintained over time. A dietitian can be very helpful in managing the weight issues associated with treatment of CD. If a patient remains underweight despite complying with the diet, the dietician may recommend gluten-free nutritional supplements.

Finally, dietitians can make sure that your restricted diet is balanced appropriately. There are three major types of nutrients: fats, carbohydrates (sugars), and protein. All three types should be eaten regularly, with a goal of having 30 percent or less of calories as fats. Gluten-containing foods tend to be carbohydrates (such as breads and pasta), so avoidance of these foods can lead to an imbalanced diet in which a large portion of the calories come from fat. This results in poor nutrition and can fuel weight gain. A dietitian can assist you with making good food choices and can recommend appropriate vitamin and mineral supplements if you have deficiencies in these areas. Examples of supplements for patients with CD include a gluten-free multivitamin as well as calcium and vitamin D (to promote bone health).

Marye comments:

I found I got more information about which foods to purchase and which not to eat from celiac support groups. Other celiac patients and the Internet were particularly helpful to me. Calling the manufacturers of the food products that I use or prior to purchasing their products helped me, too. Sometimes manufacturers even sent me coupons for their products.

Many food products state very clearly on their packages that they are "Gluten-Free" and that the food has been processed on special machinery so that it has not been contaminated by a wheat product.

59. Which grains are safe to eat?

Gluten-free grains and starches actually outnumber gluten-containing grains. The former products are good sources of carbohydrates and can be used as substitutes for making pastas, bread products, cookies, and cakes. Many gluten-free recipes are also available online and in cookbooks.

Table 15   Safe and Allowable Grains That Are Gluten Free

Amaranth	Montina
Arrowroot	Potato starch and flour
Buckwheat	Quinoa
Chickpea	Rice
Corn	Sago
Fava	Sorghum
Flax	Soy (not soy sauce)
Flours (nuts, beans, and seeds)	Tapioca
Maise	Teff
Mesquite	Pure oats?
Millet	

Hundreds of gluten-free products made of these alternative flours and starches are sold online and in supermarkets. As mentioned in Question 56, lists of these products are available from many sources. I recommend the *CSA Gluten-Free Product Listing*, an exhaustive list of gluten-free products and sites where they can be purchased. The major drawbacks associated with these products are their higher costs and sometimes unusual taste (which may not exactly match the taste of the conventional product).

60. What if I am on a gluten-free diet but still have symptoms?

There are several reasons why patients might continue to experience symptoms after a recent diagnosis of CD and beginning the gluten-free diet. The most common cause is continued consumption of gluten, either intentionally or from an unknown source (surreptitious exposure). The continued consumption might result from a lack of understanding about which foods to avoid or simply a failure to stick to the diet. Some patients may "cheat," especially early on, as sticking to the diet is restrictive and difficult. With time, once the patient becomes more educated about the diet and what happens after a dietary indiscretion, ideally compliance will improve. Symptoms may be magnified, as generally people with CD who may have had symptoms for years start to improve with appropriate diet; if they then get a small exposure, a recurrence can be distressing.

Surreptitious consumption of gluten is a very difficult issue, as only tiny amounts may cause problems. Such an exposure can result from a failure to identify gluten-containing ingredients in food or from the presence of an unknown additive in food consumed in a restaurant. Potential sources of food contamination include sharing a toaster for your rice bread with your family, sharing butter or another spread that has been inadvertently contaminated with bread crumbs, and cooking your food in a place where gluten-containing products were prepared. In addition, nonfood items, such as cosmetics, adhesives on stamps, medications, and religious products like the communion wafer, may contain gluten. Your ability to recognize potential sources of gluten will only improve with time, education, vigilance, and reading the labels on absolutely everything you eat. Dietitians can prove invaluable in this sense, as they are trained to identify potential gaps in your diet.

In addition to deviations from the gluten-free diet, there are many other causes of ongoing symptoms of CD, particularly diarrhea and possibly weight loss. The small intestine is a relatively sterile environment and normally contains only small numbers of bacteria. Several factors control this bacterial population—for example, stomach acid and gut enzymes, which aid in digestion and kill bacteria, as well as the movement or flow of nutrients from north to south, which helps to flush the bacteria downstream. In CD, this clearance system breaks down and the number and type of bacteria can increase, resulting in bacterial overgrowth. Bacterial overgrowth commonly occurs in CD but is not exclusive to CD. Symptoms of bacterial overgrowth include diarrhea, weight loss, and vitamin deficiencies. Sound familiar? It can be very difficult to tell the difference between CD and bacterial overgrowth especially when both occur at the same time. Luckily, bacterial overgrowth is easy to diagnose and treat. Treatment, which usually involves a couple of weeks of antibiotics, should be considered if the person has ongoing symptoms and his or her diet has been confirmed to be gluten free.

Microscopic colitis is a diarrheal illness that frequently accompanies CD. This inflammation of the lining of the colon or large intestine can be confirmed by biopsy. If a person has both CD and microscopic colitis, the initial treatment is a gluten-free diet, which generally resolves the colitis. Sometimes, however, the colitis may require medication for treatment. Most symptoms are controlled with one of two antidiarrheal medications: Imodium (an over-the-counter drug) or lomotil (available by prescription). On rare occasions, other medications are needed; in such a case, the issue should be managed by a gastroenterologist.

Microscopic colitis, bacterial overgrowth, and gluten contamination are generally early problems complicating CD. Symptoms may also recur after years of faithfully following the gluten-free diet. The most common cause of this problem is an unknown source of gluten in the diet, which may be easy to diagnose but hard to find. Patients on a 100 percent gluten-free diet will no longer have positive antibody testing but rather revert to negative AGA, EMA, and tTG tests. Thus, if the tests have been negative for years only to become positive now and the patient has symptoms, then gluten is the cause of the recurrence. The challenge in this case is finding the source of the gluten. In my practice, I typically send these patients back to the dietitian for a careful review of the diet. If this does not work, I may send them to an expert dietitian for a second opinion.

Any return of symptoms, particularly weight loss, years after being on the gluten-free diet is a concern and should prompt a doctor's visit. Complications of CD such as refractory sprue, ulcerative jejunitis, and small bowel lymphoma can occur late in the disease. Refractory sprue is CD that no longer responds to the diet; it may require medications such as steroids or other drugs that suppress the immune system for treatment. All three entities may actually be variations on the same CD complication, and all are serious problems that may result in severe weight loss, diarrhea, malabsorption, and even death. My recommendation is that any patient with stable CD who is compliant with the diet and who experiences new weight loss should see a gastroenterologist promptly for evaluation. Complications of CD will be addressed in detail in Part 9 of this book.

Marye comments:

I have been on a gluten-free diet for six months. I am very careful about what I eat, yet I still do have symptoms.

61. Can I eat oats?

Clearly wheat, rye, and barley contain gluten and are toxic to people with CD. The inclusion of **oats** in a gluten-free diet is the subject of much debate, however. Most oat preparations are contaminated in processing. Grains require milling prior to their use in foods, and frequently oats are milled in the same processing plants in which other grains are milled. This results in small amounts of wheat or barley entering the oats production process—which is enough to cause an immune reaction in patients.

Studies have shown that pure, uncontaminated oats, when consumed in limited amounts, are generally tolerated by adults and children and do not produce symptoms. Studies also show that patients with treated CD do not have increased blood antibodies or inflammation on small bowel biopsy after exposure to pure oats.

Historically, uncontaminated oats were not readily available in the United States, and in response celiac support groups have not recommended their use. More recently, pure oat preparations have become commercially available. The CSA gluten-free product listing recommends the products offered by Great Northern Growers located in Montana (www.greatnortherngrowers.com) and Gluten-Free Oats in Wyoming (www.glutenfreeoats.com). Both firms' products contain fewer than three parts gluten per million parts product and are likely safe. In Canada, Cream Hill Estates (www.creamhillestates.com) produces uncontaminated oats at an even higher purity standard.

Even with these low levels of contamination, some studies suggest that limited numbers of celiac patients will react to oats. Most celiac organizations and specialty medical groups allow limited consumption of pure oats. The amount of oats allowed varies between groups and ranges from ½ to 1 cup per day for adults to about ¼ cup per day for children. The general guideline is that no oats should be consumed early in the gluten-free diet. After a few months of following a strict diet, once symptoms have resolved and antibody blood testing becomes negative, small amounts of pure oats may be added into the diet and consumption advanced until the limit is reached. Some groups advocate repeat blood testing to see if the oats are prompting an immune response. Before adding oats into your diet, you should discuss this issue with your doctor and dietitian.

Marye comments:

I don't eat oats as I still have reactions to some food that I eat, even though I am very careful about my food choices. I am very careful when cooking that I use only certain utensils for stirring my food and do not touch the other food with those utensils.

62. Are there celiac-friendly stores and food manufacturers?

Given the fact that CD affects about 1 in 100 consumers, many food manufacturers and markets have begun to specialize in gluten-free products. Many supermarket chains have gluten-free sections or clearly labeled celiac-friendly products. An extensive list of celiac-friendly markets, broken down by city and state location, is available in the *CSA Gluten-Free Product Listing* (www.csaceliacs.org). Chain stores such as Albertsons, Savon, Trader Joe's, Whole Foods Markets, Shaw's, Acme, HyVee, Hannaford, Meijer Store, Jewel, and Osco also make a point of catering to those on a gluten-free diet.

Gluten-free products are available from a variety of Internet-based vendors, and a quick search will turn up many viable options. The *CSA Gluten-Free Product Listing* also includes many gluten-free vendors and producers.

Table 16   Selected Vendors of Gluten-Free Foods

Amazing Grains	Baking products	www.amazinggrains.com
Authentic Foods	Baking products	www.authenticfoods.com
Bob's Red Mill	Flours	www.bobsredmill.com
Comfy Cuisine	Prepared foods	www.comfycuisine.com
Ener-G Foods	Baked goods, pastas	www.ener-g.com
EnviroKidz	Cereals, bars, cookies	www.naturespath.com
EssenSmart Cookies	Cookies	www.essensmart.com
Food for Life Baking	Breads	www.food-for-life.com
Glutino	Baked products	www.glutino.com
Madwoman Foods	Gourmet cakes	www.madwomenfoods.com
Miss Roben's	Mixes	www.allergygrocer.com
Northern Quinoa Co.	Grains	www.quinoa.com
Pamela's Products	Mixes, cookies	www.pamelasproducts.com
Pastariso	Pastas	www.maplegrovefoods.com
Rampo Valley Brewery	Lager	www.rampovalleybrewery.com
Schar	Baked goods	www.schar.com
Sterk's Bakery	Baked goods	www.sterksbakery.com
The Teff Company	Teff grains	www.teffco.com
Twin Valley Mills	Sorghum grains	www.twinvaleymills.com

Marye comments:

There are many celiac-friendly stores and food manufacturers. A few major supermarkets have special sections devoted to celiac foods. Health food stores also have quite a selection of fresh, frozen, and packaged food products. The one thing I can't adapt to is the fresh or frozen gluten-free bread.

63. Can I drink alcohol?

Some patients with gastrointestinal conditions do not tolerate alcohol, which may also be the case for some individuals with CD. All alcohol consumed by such persons must be gluten free, so the obvious mandate is to avoid beer, ales, malts, and grain-based alcohols. Preservatives, additives, and flavorings should be avoided, and all labels must be carefully examined to identify possibly unsafe ingredients.

Table 17   Selected Producers of Gluten-Free Alcohol Products

Albertson's Corporate Brands
Anheuser-Busch
Bacardi Brands
Bard's Tale Beers
Cold Creek Distillery
Ernest and Julio Gallo
Lakefront Brewery
Ramapo Valley Brewery
Sandstone Gourmet
Trader Joe's West

Clearly, many alcoholic beverages are not made with toxic grains, leaving a wide variety to choose from aside from this brief list. Potato vodkas, light rums, and tequilas without additives are safe. Most grape-based products, such as wines, champagnes, and ports, are allowed. Rice wine or sake without additives is also safe.

Beer is a staple for many Americans, and many brewers—small and large—have produced gluten-free beer to meet this demand. Historically, small brewers (or microbrewers) such as Ramapo Valley Brewery and Lakefront Brewery have produced gluten-free beer. More recently, the giant beer maker Anheuser-Busch began brewing a gluten-free beer called Redbridge, in which sorghum is substituted for the traditional barley.

Celiac.com has a downloadable list of gluten-free drinks that can be found at www.celiac.com/st_prod.html?p_prodid=271. The Gluten Free Kitchen, Cooking with Lucy (http://gfkitchen. server101.com/GFAlcohol.htm#Wine), has a very specific list of gluten-free beverages, including wines, beers, ales, champagne, rums, tequilas, and vodkas. It is the most comprehensive and largest list I have found to date. Clan Thompson's celiac site (www.clanthompson.com/res_contacts_shop.php3) sells a variety of interesting-looking gluten-free beers as well as gluten-free guides for alcohol, medicines, and restaurants.

Marye comments:

Wine is a good option [if you want to drink alcohol]. Certain beers are also advertised as gluten free. I have gotten mixed reviews from celiac patients about alcohol. Some have told me that they have had no reaction to whisky, scotch, rye, or other liquors. Others have had a reaction—or maybe they have drunk too much alcohol in a short period of time!

64. Are there celiac-friendly restaurants? Can I eat out?

One of the most important aspects of safe dining out is the education both of yourself and of your server. It is important to understand which foods are safe and which may contain gluten, and to scrupulously avoid those gluten-containing foods.

Table 18   Prepared and Restaurant Additives That May Contain Gluten

French fry oil
Soy sauce
Teriyaki sauce
Certain salad dressings
Bacon bits
Certain mashed potato mixes
Imitation crabmeat or seafood
Meat marinade
Food additives not listed on the menu

You need to communicate clearly to your server that you have a food allergy, that you are on a special diet, and that if you eat gluten you will get sick. Most restaurant workers do not know the ingredients in the food they serve, nor do they know what gluten is. Do not hesitate to ask to speak with the manager or the chef, or check the restaurant's website prior to your visit. Also, you might call ahead to inquire about your options. Being a repeat customer may help to educate the food staff and preparers on the concept of gluten-free foods or increase their sensitivity to individuals with food allergies. Finally, if all else fails, do not hesitate to send foods back to the kitchen or leave the restaurant rather than take the risk of getting sick.

Eating out is a staple of American life, but this simple pleasure is all too often taken for granted. People newly diagnosed with CD have to undertake the difficult educational process of becoming gluten free. Part of this task is learning which restaurants have gluten-free menus or are "friendly" to individuals with food allergies or sensitivities. The Internet can prove invaluable in this way, as a quick search for "gluten-free menu" will produce thousands of hits. Many restaurants understand that their patrons may have food sensitivities and have created special gluten-free, dairy-free, or nut-free menus. Some of these options are listed on the main restaurant menu, others need to be requested from the server, and still others may be available only on the restaurant's website. Many celiac websites and support groups list "celiac-friendly" restaurants, and a variety of gluten-free restaurant guides are available.

Celiac-friendly restaurants really fall into three categories:

- Restaurants with a gluten-free menu
- Restaurants with recommendations of gluten-free foods that may be part of the regular menu
- Restaurants that simply list all of the ingredients in their meals, allowing patrons to choose which they can eat

The list in Table 19 was prepared from a careful web search and includes all three types of restaurants. Most national restaurant chains also maintain websites that list their prepared

Table 19   Selected Celiac-Friendly Restaurants Identified Through a Web Search*

Adobo Grill (Chicago)	www.adobogrill.com/oldtown/menu. aspx?s=65
Arby's	www.arbys.com/nutrition/calculator. php?mid=1&type=allergens
Ben and Jerry's	www.benandjerrys.com/our_products/ nutritional_info_all.cfm#
Biaggi's	www.biaggis.com/restaurants.htm
Bone Fish Grill	www.bonefishgrill.com/home.asp
Boston Market	www.bostonmarket.com/home
Bugaboo Creek	www.bugaboocreeksteakhouse.com/ Menu.pdf
Burger King	www.bk.com/#menu=3,2,-1
Carrabbas Italian Grill	www.carrabbas.com
Chick-fil-a	www.chickfila.com/gluten.asp
Chili's	www.gfutah.org/restaurant/Chilis.htm
Claim Jumper	www.claimjumper.com/hypertext/menu_ diet_gluten.htm
Cold Stone Cremery	www.coldstonecreamery.com/sitemap.html
Charlie Brown's Steakhouse	www.charliebrowns.com
Dairy Queen	www.dairyqueen.com/en-US/Menus+ and+Nutrition/Special+Dietary+Needs/ Gluten-Free+Products.htm
Denny's	www.dennys.com/en/cms/ Nutrition%2FAllergens/23.html
Flemming's Steakhouse	www.flemingssteakhouse.com
Jack-in-the-Box	www.jackinthebox.com/ourfood/ ingredients.php
Legal Seafood	www.legalseafoods.com/index.cfm/page/ Restaurants-now-offering-gluten-free- food/cdid/13480/pid/11282
McDonalds	www.mcdonalds.com/app_controller. nutrition.categories.gluten.index.html

Mimi's Café (Utah)	www.mimiscafe.com/
Mitchell's Fish Market	www.mitchellsfishmarket.com/index.cfm
Old Spaghetti Factory	www.osf.com/menu/location-menus/ generic_west_coast_dinner.htm
On the Border	www.ontheborder.com/menu/default.asp
Outback Steakhouse	www.outback.com/ourmenu/pdf/ glutenfree.pdf
Panera Bread	www.panerabread.com/
Pei Wei Asian Diner	www.peiwei.com/glutenfreeMenu.jsp
P.F. Changs	www.pfchangs.com/cuisine/
Ruth's Chris Steakhouse	www.ruthschris.com/
Subway	http://subway.com/subwayroot/ MenuNutrition/Nutrition/pdf/ AllergenChart.pdf
Taco Bell	www.yum.com/nutrition/documents/ tb_ingredient_statement.pdf
Taco del Mar (Utah)	www.tacodelmar.com/food/gluten.html
Ted's Montana Grill	http://tedsmontanagrill.com/nutrition_ gluten_free.html
TCBY	www.tcby.com/
Triumph Dining Guide	www.triumphdining.com/
Uno's Chicago Grill	http://unos.com/kiosk/nutritionUnos. html
Vinci (Chicago)	www.vincichicago.com/menu.aspx?s=62
Wendy's	www.wendys.com/food/pdf/us/gluten_ free_list.pdf
Wolfgang Puck	www.wolfgangpuck.com/
Wildfire (Chicago)	www.wildfirerestaurant.com/second_level/ menu/celiac.htm
Z Tejas Grill	www.ztejas.com/menu.php?section=menu

* Many other national chains and local restaurants have gluten-free selections, so you should do further research in your area.

foods' ingredients; if you have questions about a particular menu option, you can easily check these sites.

When eating out, educating your server is key to avoiding a gluten-containing or -contaminated meal. Many support groups and authors recommend the use of educational cards. These cards, which explain what CD is and which foods and grains need to be avoided, can be provided to restaurant servers if questions arise. These cards are generally available in many languages, and books and websites offer various types of cards. The website www.celiactravel.com/restaurant-cards. html, for example, offers free educational dining out cards in 38 different languages. A small donation is suggested by the website but payment is voluntary.

Marye comments:

A few chain restaurants have gluten-free menus. I have also found that when I explain my allergy to wheat/gluten, restaurant owners and staff will become very creative and offer or suggest different ways of preparing food that you can eat. They seem to take a certain pride in meeting the challenge.

65. What are some sources of gluten contamination?

Gluten is everywhere, and avoiding it is akin to negotiating a minefield. Gluten contamination can generally be classified into two categories: (1) environmental and nondietary sources and (2) food associated.

Environmental and Nondietary Gluten

Sharing cooking utensils or kitchens can result in food contamination. For example, rice bread toasted in a toaster that is used by other family members can be a source of gluten contamination. Similarly, sharing kitchen utensils or preparation surfaces can result in contamination of food. For example, preparing rice pasta and regular pasta at the same time and sharing the boiling water, bowls, or a colander may lead to cross-contamination. Likewise, some restaurants prepare broiled meats on bread and then discard the bread. All of these are examples food being contaminated by the environment.

Other nondietary sources of gluten are beauty aids. For example, some lipsticks and facial products contain gluten proteins.

Some pills and medications, whether prescribed or available over the counter, and even some supplements, are produced with gluten binders. If you have questions about a particular medication, you should ask your pharmacist, contact the drug's manufacturer, or check the associated website. Many lists of gluten-free medications are available on the Internet and from celiac support groups.

Gluten is a sticky protein when wet, and because of this property it can be used as glue. Gluten may be present in the adhesive on envelopes and stamps, such that licking a stamp or an envelope can result in contamination. Gluten is also found in communion wafers, which presents another source of nondietary exposure.

Dietary Gluten

If you have CD, you must read all labels of everything, as gluten is present in all kinds of food products besides the obvious bread and pasta. Ongoing CD symptoms despite a 100 percent gluten-free diet, a phenomenon called surreptitious gluten consumption, generally results from an unknown source of gluten ingestion despite being knowingly faithful with your diet.

Always read the label. Become educated so that you know how to look for items that may contain wheat derivatives, extracts, or contaminants. For example, some grains that are safe to eat may nevertheless be milled in the same plants or by the same machines that mill wheat products, resulting in a contamination of an apparently safe product. I am always highly impressed by how educated and "connected" my celiac patients are; thanks to their continuous educational process in investigating the gluten-free diet, much of this information about safe foods is widely available and you do not have to "reinvent the wheel." Instead, you can turn to support groups run by those with CD, medical websites, and the many books and publications listing safe or unsafe foods.

Reading the label is a benefit if you are looking for the obvious, such as wheat. *All* potentially toxic additives need to be identified, however, so you need to learn how to detect possible gluten-containing ingredients. Be aware of toxic grains, including the different species of wheat, as they are not obvi-

Table 20   Possible Gluten-Containing Food Additives

Artificial and natural flavors
Baker's or brewers yeast
Dextrin
Caramel coloring
Hydrolyzed plant, vegetable, natural protein
Malt
Maltodextrin
Modified starch or starch
Soy sauce (not soy bean products)
Vinegar

Table 21   A Limited List of Possibly Contaminated Foods

McDonalds French fry oil
Baked beans
Soy sauce
Dried fruits
Teriyaki sauce
Seasoned nuts
Malted milk
Certain salad dressings
Bacon bits
Certain mashed potato mixes and rice mixes
Cheese foods or spreads
Prepared meats or hot dogs
Imitation crabmeat or seafood
Meat marinades or extenders
Some ice creams

ous like those listed in Question 55. A good patient guide like the *CSA Gluten-Free Product Listing* can also be very helpful understanding which products are safe or contain gluten.

Marye comments:

[Gluten contamination can be avoided by] using separate utensils when cooking for yourself. Try not to kiss someone on the lips who has eaten wheat, grain, or oat products.

66. What about the communion wafer and other gluten-containing religious products?

First, a disclaimer: I am not Catholic, but I have found wheat-containing products and religion to be a complicated and fascinating issue. The relationships among CD; individuals of Irish, Italian, and French Canadian heritage; and Catholicism have been a great subject of debate in the press, among religious scholars and on celiac websites. In my practice, I have treated a number of patients, including clergy members, who have CD and who face issues with Catholic communion.

"Spiritual communion" is an act expressing what was described by St. Thomas Aquinas "as an ardent desire to receive Jesus in the Most Holy Sacrament and in lovingly embracing Him." Spiritual communion is always available and might be especially appropriate when traveling or attending Mass outside your parish. (Adapted from information about Catholic communion and celiac disease from the Catholic Celiac Society)

At the Last Supper, Jesus gave his disciples bread and wine and said, "Do this in memory of me." Accordingly, canon law and the Roman Catholic Church state that during communion, the **host** (wafer) must be made of wheat and water and that the wine must be made from grape juice. Pastoral guidelines state that "Church teaching has no authority to change what Christ instituted." This presents a problem to patients with CD and can be a source of either known or unknown gluten in the diet from the communion wafer.

Host

The wheat-containing wafer taken at communion to symbolize Christ.

The issue of a gluten-free host or rice-based host was addressed in 2003 by then-Cardinal Joseph Ratzinger (now Pope Benedict XVI), in a letter to the Presidents of Conferences of Bishops: "It is impossible to consecrate a host made of something other than wheat. No priest or bishop can change this longstanding teaching of the Catholic Church. Hosts that are completely gluten-free are invalid matter for the celebration of the Eucharist." This policy has resulted in the denial of or invalidation of communion, particularly in the first communion of children with CD, because of the use of a gluten-free host or the inability to take a gluten-containing host.

Fermentum

The material added to grape juice to make religious consecrated wine. It may contain gluten.

Consecrated wine from the priest's chalice may be contaminated by the **fermentum,** a small piece of the wheat-containing host that is added to the wine during the consecration. Consecrated wine can also be contaminated by other parishioners who have taken the host and drank from the chalice. This issue should be discussed with your priest, as it may be possible to use a chalice that is reserved for use only by individuals with CD and is gluten free.

Low-gluten host

A modified communion wafer that contains a small amount of gluten.

There is some debate in the literature as to whether any amount of gluten is safe for celiacs. Because of this controversy, alternatives to the conventional host have become available in the form of a **low-gluten host.** One low-gluten host approved by the Catholic Church is produced by the Benedictine Sisters of Clyde (www.benedictinesisters.org; 800-223-2772). This host contains the minimum amount of gluten needed to obtain church approval and is less than 0.01 percent gluten by weight. To take communion, one does not need to consume the entire wafer—one fourth of the wafer is enough—which can reduce gluten ingestion further. Low-gluten hosts should be placed in a clean **pyx** (the container used to carry the host).

Pyx

The vessel used to store the wafer host in communion.

The University of Chicago Celiac Disease Program (www.celiacdisease.net) has proposed the following guidelines for those taking the low-gluten host:

- See your doctor and obtain follow-up blood testing for CD with a tTG or EMA test. When these tests are negative on a gluten-free diet, then a low-gluten host can be used. If the tests are positive, then the low-gluten host should not be used.
- Book a return appointment for repeat testing in six months after starting the low-gluten host.
- Have repeat testing done to see whether the results of the antibody tests have changed. If they remain negative or low, then it is probably safe to continue the low-gluten host. If the levels increase, then the culprit may be the host or another gluten contaminant in the diet.

There are many resources available regarding the issue of communion and CD. An excellent patient information flier is available from the Catholic Celiac Society at www.catholicceliacs. org. Pastoral guidelines for the use of low-gluten hosts are available at www.dow.org/documents/CeliacGUIDELINES.doc. Permission to use the low-gluten host may be required, and the necessary form is available at www.rcab.org/OfficeForWorship/ PastoralNotes/CeliacWorship.html. Celiac support groups and the Internet are also terrific resources.

Marye comments:

I have stopped receiving communion.

67. I have symptoms. Should I just have a trial of a gluten-free diet?

Patients frequently ask if they should try a restricted diet. In my practice, I do not recommend trials of a gluten-free diet. There are several reasons for this reluctance, but the most important question is: What are we treating? If there is a concern that a patient has CD, then appropriate blood testing and confirmatory endoscopy and biopsy, if needed, are in order. A limited diet is the wrong approach, because many people who actually have irritable bowel syndrome (IBS) rather than CD will improve with such dietary changes.

Another reason to avoid dietary trials is the fact they are not uniform or consistent. Patients who try a gluten-free diet frequently avoid just the obvious sources of gluten—breads, pastas, and wheat-containing products. They typically do not maintain strict adherence to the diet by reading labels and avoiding contamination of food. Instead, they might get some limited information or find something on the Internet and try it. Generally, these patients have not seen a dietitian and really do not understand the finer points of the dietary restrictions necessary. As discussed in Question 58, patients with true CD need to go through an educational process that includes follow-up and evaluation by a dietitian.

In my own practice, I have seen referred patients who have been told by their primary healthcare providers to try the diet. I strongly disagree with this approach, predominantly for the reasons already discussed. Antibody testing and small intestinal biopsies need to be done while the patient is on a gluten-containing diet. If the patient is on a strict gluten-free diet, then the testing will produce false-negative results (negative test results when the patient actually has CD) and the appropriate diagnosis will be missed. Generally, I suggest to these patients that they should resume a "normal" diet and come back in about two months for testing, as it takes several weeks for the body to have a detectable immune response.

68. Does a gluten-free diet help irritable bowel syndrome?

Irritable bowel syndrome (IBS) is a condition characterized by diarrhea and/or constipation associated with abdominal discomfort that lasts for a period of three months or longer. Generally, the discomfort improves after a bowel movement. Treatment for IBS includes restriction of the diet. Foods whose consumption is to be limited include caffeine, spicy foods, chocolate, dairy products, fatty foods, and possibly gluten. Not all of these foods need to be limited, so to some extent treatment is a trial process to see which foods the particular individual should avoid.

In such cases, patients do not have true food allergies, but rather food sensitivities. This is an important distinction. An allergy is an inflammatory response by the immune system to a foreign substance or protein. With this inflammation comes damage, which requires a period of repair or healing. Sensitivity, by contrast, is intolerance to food; there is no inflammation. For example, a person might experience cramps and diarrhea after eating a creamy or fatty meal. If you have a food sensitivity, once the offending food is out of your system, there is no damage or long-term consequences.

Some patients with IBS (without CD) do respond to a gluten-restricted diet. As mentioned earlier, gluten is difficult to digest. Because individuals with IBS have sensitive gastrointestinal systems, they may develop symptoms with gluten ingestion. This is not an immune system process for these patients, however, unlike the inflammation experienced by individuals with CD. Usually a gluten-free diet is not needed in case of IBS, only a low-gluten diet. Food sensitivities have a volume or amount factor, meaning that small amounts of problematic foods can usually be tolerated. Thus, for gluten-sensitive IBS patients, avoidance of bread, pastas, and cereals may be helpful. A strict gluten-free diet with label reading and complete restriction of all dietary gluten is generally unnecessary.

PART SIX

Management of Celiac Disease

Do I need to stay on a gluten-free diet for life?

What's next if the diet is not working?

Do I need any vaccinations?

More . . .

69. Do I need to stay on a gluten-free diet for life?

Therapy for CD consists of a lifelong gluten-free diet. Adult CD does not go away with a gluten-free diet—it just goes into remission. With a strict diet, the results of blood testing (that is, the AGA, EMA, and tTG) become negative and can be used to determine whether a patient is truly gluten free. Likewise, small bowel biopsies will improve and may return to normal when a person faithfully follows the diet. Despite these normal findings, CD is still present. Thus, if gluten is added back into the diet, symptoms will return, as will the markers of the disease.

Strict adherence to the gluten-free diet is particularly difficult for asymptomatic patients, as these individuals do not develop overt physical symptoms with gluten consumption. It is likely easier to stick with the diet when a patient has cramps, gas, and diarrhea and generally feels lousy after eating gluten. This direct relationship creates a positive reinforcement promoting dietary compliance in symptomatic patients. A similar reinforcement may not occur in persons with silent disease and makes staying on the diet more difficult.

Aside from the improvement in symptoms, the major reason to stay on the diet faithfully is the prevention of celiac-associated complications. Nutritional deficiencies are corrected with dietary compliance but will recur with food indiscretion. Iron and vitamin B_{12} deficiency, which may be manifested as anemia, difficulty walking, or numbness in the hands and feet, can occur years after resuming gluten consumption. Osteoporosis from vitamin D deficiency takes years to occur and similarly may be discovered late after stopping the diet. Staying with the diet also improves body composition, as a person's body mass index (BMI), weight, fat mass, and bone mineral density all improve with sustained adherence to a gluten-free diet.

Refractory sprue is characterized by diarrhea, weight loss, and vitamin deficiencies that persist despite compliance with a strict gluten-free diet. The risk of CD becoming refractory may be increased with dietary indiscretion. Major complications of CD include lymphoma (a cancer affecting the lymph nodes) and death; these risks are increased in people with CD compared to those without CD. The risk of death for patients with CD compared to the normal population is even greater if they do not stay with the diet, with the excess risk of death usually being related to the increased cancer risk and ongoing malabsorption of nutrients. Thankfully, the overall excess death risk in CD is low and can be brought even lower by lifelong compliance with a gluten-free diet.

Studies demonstrate a clear benefit for those patients who stick with the diet. One study of CD patients showed a more than 50 percent reduction in the lymphoma risk for those who followed a strict diet. Another study demonstrated that patients with CD on a strict diet had no increased risk of cancer compared to members of a control group without CD. A study of patients with dermatitis herpetiformis revealed that those who developed lymphoma were more likely not to be compliant with a strict gluten-free diet.

One reassuring note is the fact that the overall risk of cancer in CD is low regardless of diet. One study calculated that 120 cases of lymphoma occurred in 100,000 patient-years of disease. Another way to look at this statistic is to say that 120 cases of lymphoma occurred in 10,000 celiac patients who were followed for 10 years.

Some children have experienced a variant of CD called latent CD. These children had CD, went on a gluten-free diet, and completely recovered. As either older children or adults, they were then able to tolerate a gluten-containing diet without symptoms. This small celiac patient population may be the only group who can go off the diet. It is unclear what the

Management of Celiac Disease

long-term issues are for this small group, but sometimes they may redevelop symptoms, requiring that they return to the gluten-free diet.

Marye comments:

Why wouldn't you stay on the gluten-free diet? Once you start asking questions about the foods you are about to eat, you educate yourself on the products and foods that you need to avoid. It is so simple to stick to a gluten-free diet.

70. Can I ever eat any gluten-containing foods? If I do, what will happen?

Gluten is toxic to people with CD and should be avoided by them. Frequently, patients state they are on the diet but have indiscretions or knowingly eat gluten. Many patients may not recognize the nonfood sources of gluten and, therefore, continue to eat gluten despite apparent compliance with the diet. Not all patients with CD are willing to go gluten free, so they continue to follow a regular diet and have symptoms. Continued gluten ingestion stimulates an immune response of inflammation within the small intestine and antibody production, which results in intestinal damage and prevents healing.

Patients who were symptomatic with bloating, diarrhea, pain, and weight loss before beginning a gluten-free diet will have symptoms with a gluten exposure after starting the diet. As an example, in my practice, a patient was referred to me for evaluation. The referring doctor did blood testing, with the tTG test being positive, and suggested the patient start the diet. During my meeting with the patient, I recommended resumption of gluten, as this is required to get a positive biopsy. Within a few days of returning to a normal diet, she was miserable, having abdominal pain, diarrhea, and severe crippling fatigue, and just felt sick. The patient refused to continue gluten consumption and, after several weeks of resuming the gluten-free diet, felt better. This is an extreme example but a good illustration. Usually, patients develop symptoms that may take several days to weeks to improve, because the inflammatory damage to the small intestine takes some time to heal. Although most patients have a milder reaction to gluten, there is a wide range in their responses—from no symptoms to severe problems.

Patients who are asymptomatic may tolerate gluten without symptoms yet still have an immune response to the gluten. This phenomenon prevents resolution of the damage and inflammation of the intestine and allows for progression of the disease. Periodic gluten ingestion does not protect against the complications of CD even in asymptomatic patients. These patients are at increased risk of vitamin deficiencies, osteoporosis, malabsorption, and cancer. Interestingly, some asymptomatic patients with CD may improve with adherence to a strict diet and then have a feeling of illness after eating gluten. It is likely that these patients have had mild illness for so long that they did not appreciate how poorly they felt until they were reexposed to gluten.

Unappreciated or unknown gluten ingestion is the most common reason for lack of improvement of symptoms. When a patient with a new diagnosis of CD goes on the gluten-free diet and continues to have symptoms, the first move is to send the individual back to the dietitian for reevaluation and review of the diet. Likewise, if a patient has been on a gluten-free diet for years and suddenly has a recurrence of symptoms, a dietitian evaluation is needed to check the diet.

Some patients knowingly eat gluten and live with the results. I have several patients who periodically consume bread, pizza, pasta, or beer because they "have to" or because they want to go out with friends and be "normal." Others cannot afford to go completely gluten free because the rice bread is so expensive. These patients generally develop symptoms when they eat gluten but are willing to suffer the consequences. They

Management of Celiac Disease

are sick for a few days and then recover with a return to the appropriate diet. This pattern reinforces the importance of sticking to the diet, as patients can clearly see the relationship between gluten consumption and their illness.

The most difficult group of patients to treat includes those who are sick with diarrhea, weight loss, and malabsorption, yet will not stay on a gluten-free diet. As mentioned in Question 9, there is an association between CD and psychiatric illness. Sometimes patients do not have the capacity to understand the diet or recognize the need to follow it faithfully. These patients may develop severe malabsorption with extreme weight loss, dehydration, and vitamin deficiencies, leading to hospitalization and (rarely) death.

71. What's next if the diet is not working?

The gluten-free diet is very effective as a treatment for CD. If a patient with CD is on the diet and still has symptoms, then usually there is a problem with the diet, and gluten is sneaking in somehow. An easy way to confirm this suspicion is with repeat antibody blood testing. With time and a strict diet, the antibody levels will drop, ultimately becoming negative. If this change does not occur, then most likely the patient's diet includes some form of gluten.

If my patients have continued positive blood work, then I send them back to the dietitian for a careful review of the diet, focusing on gluten contamination of food or other unknown gluten sources. Examples include foods contaminated by family members who are sharing butter, jam, or jelly and "double dipping" a knife that has been used on regular bread, with tiny crumbs getting into the product. Sharing a toaster with others might also lead to contamination, with crumbs of the regular bread being transferred to the rice bread. Other gluten sources that may be difficult to find include taking communion, licking envelopes, and using gluten-containing cosmetics or medications.

Once the possibility of gluten entering the diet has been excluded, several other explanations for ongoing symptoms must be considered. Consumption of dairy products in the setting of lactose intolerance (a condition that is often found in conjunction with CD) will result in cramps, gas, and diarrhea. Bacterial overgrowth is also common in persons with CD and will cause weight loss, anemia, and diarrhea. Microscopic colitis, which likewise occurs frequently in CD, will cause severe watery diarrhea. Evaluation for these entities needs to be done because these conditions are often present when CD is diagnosed, and all are easy to treat.

Still other possibilities exist as rationales for continued celiac symptoms. The diagnosis of CD may be wrong: Not all villous atrophy is CD, and other diseases should be considered by your doctor, particularly if celiac blood testing results are negative. Refractory sprue consists of atrophy of the small intestinal villi that produces positive blood tests and malabsorption that does not respond to the diet. This disease can be difficult to treat and requires medications that suppress the immune system, such as steroids. Two notable complications of CD, ulcerative jejunitis and lymphoma, will present with recurrent celiac symptoms of diarrhea, weight loss, and possibly night-time sweating. If a patient with CD has ongoing weight loss or recurrent weight loss after years of following a strict gluten-free diet, this is an ominous sign that requires prompt evaluation by the physician.

72. Are there any other foods that may need to be avoided aside from those with gluten?

The small intestine is the site for digestion and absorption of food and nutrients. Diseases of the small intestine such as CD cause damage, resulting in abnormal digestion and impaired absorption. Some foods that are affected by this process should probably be avoided early on after the initial diagnosis, which allows for intestinal healing with the gluten-free diet. These foods can then be added back to the diet over time.

Dairy products such as milk contain a sugar called lactose. Lactose is digested by lactase, an enzyme that is present in the intestinal villi. Damage to the villi impairs production of lactase, leading to lactose intolerance. Frequently, eating dairy products or drinking milk will cause diarrhea, gas, bloating, and cramps in patients who are starting the gluten-free diet. This problem usually resolves after a few months on the diet, and dairy products can then be added back to the diet.

There is a great deal of overlap between the symptoms of CD and the symptoms of irritable bowel syndrome. Patients with IBS have several food sensitivities, so avoidance of these foods might reduce some CD symptoms. These foods do not have to be strictly eliminated in a person with CD (the person does not have a true food allergy), but their avoidance may improve diarrhea, bloating, and cramps. Limitation of caffeine, alcohol, fatty foods, spicy foods, and chocolate may also improve symptoms in some patients. Again, this is not a strict recommendation in the same way that gluten avoidance is mandatory; it is merely a suggestion for those with food-related symptoms.

73. What should the doctor be following?

The issue here is twofold: What should be checked during the initial diagnosis, and what should be followed over the long term? I am a physician educator, meaning that in addition to seeing patients I train other doctors to become gastroenterologists. The most important lesson I learned in medical school came on the first day, and now I share it with my trainees: "Listen to your patients; they will tell you what is wrong with them." I try to treat the "whole patient." Given the life-altering diagnosis of CD, your doctor should treat you similarly. This means that your doctor should address not only the medical issues directly related to CD but also any associated problems.

When making the initial diagnosis of CD, the most obvious things to watch are your symptoms and your response to the gluten-free diet. Weight is a major issue: At diagnosis, patients may be either underweight or overweight; after beginning the diet, however, most patients will gain weight from improved nutrient absorption. Thus the patient's weight fluctuations need to be monitored over time. Patients may need to return to the dietitian if they experience excessive weight gain to add a calorie restriction to the gluten-free diet. Conversely, if patients are underweight, they may need recommendations on gluten-free nutritional supplements that will help them gain weight. Other symptoms such as gas, bloating, diarrhea, and nongastrointestinal symptoms also need to be further investigated and treated if the diet does not resolve them.

Initial testing includes evaluation of anemia, liver tests, some vitamin levels, and testing for bone health. A list of recommended initial evaluations including blood testing and bone density scanning appears in Question 53. A bone density scan is an x-ray test that checks for osteoporosis. Patients should undergo such scanning at baseline and then every one to two years thereafter. This policy allows for early intervention if osteoporosis is discovered as well as follow-up to see whether any medications prescribed are working.

After making the initial diagnosis and starting patients on a gluten-free diet, I usually see my patients three to four months later, depending on their illness. Once patients are stable, all of the symptoms are resolved, and any vitamin deficiencies are corrected, I see them annually. The benefit of seeing a gastroenterologist in addition to your regular doctor is that gastroenterologists understand how to prevent and treat problems that may complicate CD. A continuing relationship with a gastroenterologist also helps when a problem arises, because you know someone to call.

Patients who have recently been diagnosed with CD need to undergo an evaluation with a registered dietitian and receive dietary teaching. At least one return visit with the dietician should be scheduled to ensure they understand the gluten-free

Table 22   Recommended Annual Testing for Patients with Celiac Disease

Complete blood count
Liver function tests
Calcium
Vitamin D level
Vitamin B$_{12}$ level
Carotene
Zinc
Bone density scan every 1 to 2 years

diet and are not having any problems. Ideally, the dietitian will provide additional resources such as information on local support groups and helpful books.

These recommendations apply to patients in the maintenance phase of CD who have few or no symptoms and are successfully complying with a strict gluten-free diet. If you have new or ongoing symptoms (particularly weight loss), you should call or visit your doctor promptly.

74. Do the antiendomysial antibody or tissue transglutaminase blood tests need to be repeated periodically?

Blood testing with an EMA or tTG usually provides a number—a level—as a result, which falls within a range from positive to negative. Positive test results correlate well with recent exposure to gluten-containing food; a negative test result means that the person has not consumed dietary gluten for several months. Thus this kind of test is a good objective gauge regarding the effectiveness of the gluten-free diet. In my practice, I perform an EMA or tTG for my patients annually to watch their diet. If the test is positive, then more education on the diet and sources of gluten contamination is recommended, along with a visit to the dietitian.

The EMA and tTG tests are particularly helpful in patients whose results are negative but who still have symptoms. In these cases, symptoms may be related to a different condition that can occur with or complicate CD. Examples include bacterial overgrowth, lactose intolerance, and microscopic colitis, all of which are treatable. Complications of CD include refractory sprue, ulcerative jejunitis, and lymphoma, which are more difficult to treat. These entities require further evaluation, including blood testing, to ensure that the patient is strictly adhering to the gluten-free diet.

Another benefit of annual testing is that it becomes possible to change the diet (such as by adding back certain foods) and determine whether the patient has an immunologic response to that change. When patients are on a gluten-free diet for a few months and the antibody testing becomes negative, then pure oats can be added to the diet in limited amounts. If the patient becomes symptomatic, then the oats are culprit and their consumption is stopped. Periodic blood testing will reveal whether there is an antibody response to the oats.

In my experience, the most important reason to do annual testing for CD is a simple one: It gives patients peace of mind to know that their diet is working.

75. What is bacterial overgrowth, and should I be checked for it?

The gut is full of bacteria, whose numbers increase the farther downstream in the gut you go. The colon is full of bacteria—mostly beneficial—that aid in digestion and even produce some vitamins such as folic acid and **vitamin K**. By contrast, the small intestine is a relatively sterile environment but does contain a small number of bacteria. Protective mechanisms that keep the bacteria level low in the small intestine include stomach acid, digestive enzymes, and movement of material, constantly flushing things into the colon.

Vitamin K
A fat-soluble vitamin made by intestinal bacteria that helps to clot blood.

In CD, this balance is disrupted. The numbers and type of bacteria can increase in the small intestine, a condition called bacterial overgrowth. Bacterial overgrowth can damage the lining of the small intestine, such that biopsies taken from people with this disorder can look similar to those seen in CD. Typically, bacterial overgrowth causes weight loss, diarrhea, gas, bloating, anemia, and vitamin deficiencies. It can be difficult to distinguish the symptoms of CD from the symptoms of bacterial overgrowth. Frequently, bacterial overgrowth can be present in untreated CD, compounding the symptoms associated with CD. Bacterial overgrowth is also a common cause of CD symptoms that occur despite adherence to a strict gluten-free diet.

Two tests are used to diagnose bacterial overgrowth, one invasive and the other noninvasive. The invasive and more sensitive test involves taking a sample of the small intestinal fluid during an endoscopy test. This fluid is sent to the lab for a culture. If the culture reveals that a certain kind or number of bacteria are present in the specimen, then the test is considered positive.

The other, noninvasive test for bacterial overgrowth is called a breath test. It is generally done in a doctor's office or at the hospital. First you drink a special sugar solution, and then your breath (a gas) is collected periodically for about two hours and analyzed. Humans normally do not produce hydrogen or methane, but the bacteria in our intestines do; their production of these gases is exhaled in the breath and can be detected. If hydrogen and methane are found in certain quantities in the breath, then the test is considered positive and bacterial overgrowth is present. The breath test is not sensitive, however, and is falsely negative in about 50 percent of tests.

Bacterial overgrowth is common following many processes that affect the small intestine, such as diabetes, Crohn's disease, small intestinal diverticulosis, advancing age, **scleroderma,** prior surgery on the intestine, and CD. I generally do not recommend the endoscopic testing to my patients,

Frequently, bacterial overgrowth can be present in untreated CD, compounding the symptoms associated with CD. Bacterial overgrowth is also a common cause of CD symptoms that occur despite adherence to a strict gluten-free diet.

Scleroderma

An autoimmune inflammatory condition that can affect any part of the body and is characterized by thickening and scarring of the affected part.

as it is invasive. By contrast, the breath test is not invasive, but if negative may actually be an inaccurate result. If I feel strongly that one of my patients has bacterial overgrowth, then I will recommend empiric treatment; in other words, I will treat the patient for this condition without testing if there is a high likelihood of bacterial overgrowth. Treatment involves taking a course of antibiotics (virtually any antibiotic will work), usually over a period of about two weeks. Many patients require retreatment or periodic antibiotics, especially if they have a structural abnormality in the small intestine (for example, caused by prior surgery) or a narrowing of the intestine (stricture). Luckily, of all the diseases that can involve the small intestine, bacterial overgrowth is easy to treat and its eradication can make a dramatic difference in improving symptoms. For this reason, I have a very low threshold for giving a short course of antibiotics to my patients to see if it helps.

76. Should I have a bone density scan?

All patients with newly diagnosed CD should definitely have a bone density scan (called DXA or DEXA scan). This test measures how much calcium and minerals are contained in the bones. This information is important because as the mineral content drops, the bones thin and the risk of incurring a fracture even with little or no trauma increases. A bone density scan can determine whether the bones are normal density, there is minor thinning (osteopenia), or there is severe thinning (osteoporosis). Both osteopenia and osteoporosis should be treated to stop bone deterioration and improve bone density.

Bone density testing can be done in some doctors' offices or in a hospital. Typically, the patient lies on a table, and a mechanical arm passes over the patient emitting low-level x-rays. The test takes about 10 minutes, and the radiation exposure is similar to that with a chest x-ray. The bone density is measured in two places—the hip and the spine—and compared to the expected normal levels for your age. The result is called a **T-score**. A T-score of greater than −1 is normal; −1 to −2.5 is osteopenia; and less than −2.5 is osteoporosis. Based on these results, your doctor can make recommendations if treatment is needed.

T-score

The scoring scale for bone density scans. It is used to diagnose osteoporosis.

Risk factors for osteoporosis include female sex, family history of osteoporosis, smoking, being thin, lack of exercise, Caucasian race, use of certain medications such as steroids, menopause, lack of regular sun exposure, low consumption of dairy products (which contain calcium and vitamin D), and diseases of the small intestine such as CD. Vitamin D and calcium absorption in the small intestine is linked to fat absorption. In CD, fat is poorly absorbed, which increases the risk of osteoporosis because the calcium and vitamin are not properly absorbed from nutrients and they are lost. Upon testing for CD, many asymptomatic patients who are found to have osteoporosis and low vitamin D levels turn out to have CD.

Risk factors for osteoporosis include female sex, family history of osteoporosis, smoking, being thin, lack of exercise, Caucasian race, use of certain medications such as steroids, menopause, lack of regular sun exposure, low consumption of dairy products, and diseases of the small intestine such as CD.

The bone density scan provides a baseline with which to compare bone density measurements taken in the future, thereby determining whether bone loss is progressing. I usually recommend bone density testing every one to two years. This testing pattern helps determine whether bone loss is still occurring, has stabilized, or is improving thanks to the use of calcium and vitamin D supplements. If the initial exam shows osteoporosis, follow-up exams can be used to measure the patient's response to medications. Medications for bone health include over-the-counter calcium and vitamin D supplements as well as a class of prescription-only drugs called **bisphosphonates,** which are available as pills or long-acting intravenous forms.

Bisphosphonates

A class of drugs that is used to treat osteoporosis.

Marye comments:

Once you are older than age 40, a bone density scan is something that should be done on a regular basis.

77. Do I need to take vitamins, minerals, or vitamin B$_{12}$ shots?

There are no recommended guidelines for vitamin or mineral supplementation for patients with CD. A variety of gluten-free vitamins and supplements are available; you can find a list of them in the *CSA Gluten-free Product Listing* (www.csaceliacs.org). A web search will also produce many hits facilitating purchase of gluten-free nutritionals.

Patients with CD should be routinely tested to check their vitamin D, vitamin B$_{12}$, beta carotene, calcium, and iron status. Your physical symptoms also might dictate other routine evaluation and supplementation. For example, muscle cramps may be related to a magnesium deficiency, and poor wound healing could result from a zinc deficiency. Both of these mineral deficiencies occur in the setting of chronic diarrhea. Numbness in the feet and legs, difficulty in position sense (for example, falling over in the shower when soap gets in your eyes), and anemia could potentially be signs of a vitamin B$_{12}$ deficiency.

Table 23   Nutrients at Risk in Patients with Celiac Disease

Nutrient	Role	Recommended Testing
Vitamin A	Eye and skin health	Carotene level
Vitamin B$_{12}$	Anemia, nerve and brain function	Yes
Vitamin D	Bone health	Yes
Calcium	Bone health, muscle, nerve function	Yes
Iron	Anemia	Complete blood count
Thiamine	Heart and brain function, beri beri	If indicated
Magnesium	Muscle function	If indicated
Zinc	Wound healing, abnormal taste	If indicted

*I routinely
recommend
a gluten-free
multivitamin,
calcium, and
vitamin D
supplements
for all of my
patients with
CD.*

I routinely recommend a gluten-free multivitamin, calcium, and vitamin D supplements for all of my patients with CD. This combination covers most of the vitamins and minerals that I would recommend to any patient with a GI-related problem. If any other deficiencies are picked up through screening or because of symptoms, they should be treated as well. A multivitamin will provide the recommended daily allotment (RDA) of most vitamins and some minerals. Vitamin and mineral levels should be rechecked annually to ensure adequate supplementation, and doses adjusted as necessary following this testing.

Marye comments:

Once I started taking vitamin D and B$_{12}$ shots, I felt better. My skin, hair, and nails improved. I also found I had less cramping and pain.

Table 24   Recommended Vitamin and Mineral Doses to Replace Vitamin Deficiencies

Nutrient	Recommended Replacement Dose
Vitamin A	Vitamin A can be toxic; replace with a carotene supplement*
Vitamin B$_{12}$	Monthly 1000 mcg intramuscular injections
Vitamin D	800iu daily; if level very low, use prescription vitamin D*
Calcium	1200 to 1800 mg a day
Iron	If low, 325 mg three a day for one month; would not use chronically without a doctor's recommendation
Thiamine	100 mg per day for acute illness, then 10 mg per day*
Magnesium	Magnesium oxide 200 to 400 mg up to twice a day*; may cause diarrhea
Zinc	Do not exceed 10 to 15 mg per day*; high doses can cause toxicity

* A multivitamin provides the daily requirements for these nutrients.

78. Do I need any vaccinations?

Celiac disease does not substantially increase the risk of infection for most patients, but certain vaccinations might be indicated. The **spleen** is an organ of the immune system that maintains immune function by making antibodies, fighting infection, and filtering the blood, thereby removing bacteria and old blood cells. It is located in the left upper part of the abdomen under the rib cage, which protects it. The spleen is about the size of a fist and is very sensitive to trauma. It is often damaged as a result of motor vehicle accidents and sports injuries. In such a case, the spleen can shatter or rupture with severe, life-threatening bleeding that requires emergency surgery to remove it.

Celiac disease can impair the function of the spleen, resulting in **hyposplenism** (an underactive spleen). People without spleens or those with hyposplenism are at increased risk of certain infections. Infection with *Pneumococcus*, a bacterium that causes pneumonia, is particularly dangerous in individuals without a spleen and can be very severe or even life-threatening. Some doctors recommend vaccination for this infection. The **pneumococcal vaccine** is a shot given roughly every five years that protects individuals only against pneumococcal pneumonia. It is not effective against many other bacteria that can cause lung infections and pneumonia. Given that patients with CD and hyposplenism are uniquely at increased risk of severe pneumococcal infection, the vaccination should be considered.

Every fall the issue of getting a **flu shot** comes up. This vaccination is recommended for children, people age 65 and older, and individuals with chronic disease. Given that CD is a chronic illness, an annual flu shot would be recommended for these patients.

There is also an association between CD and liver disease. If you have abnormal liver tests, autoimmune liver disease, or any

Spleen
An organ in the left upper part of the abdomen that protects the body against infection.

Hyposplenism
A condition in which an underactive spleen predisposes a person to certain infections.

Pneumococcal vaccine
A vaccine against a type of pneumonia.

Given that patients with CD and hyposplenism are uniquely at increased risk of severe pneumococcal infection, the vaccination should be considered.

Flu shot
An annual vaccination against the flu. It is generally recommended for chronically ill individuals, people older than age 65, and small children.

Management of Celiac Disease

151

other liver abnormality, then you should be tested for hepatitis A and B. This measure is suggested to rule out an active
or prior infection; a negative test result means that you have
never been exposed to these viruses. Persons with underlying
liver disease are at increased risk of developing severe hepatitis
if they acquire a hepatitis A or B infection. Thus vaccination
should be considered for both viruses if testing is negative.

You should discuss the issue of vaccinations with your healthcare provider. This discussion will ensure that you have been
properly vaccinated and that all of your vaccinations are up-
to-date (some, such as the tetanus vaccination, may require
periodic "booster shots").

79. Should I take supplements such as fish oil or probiotics?

Currently, there are no formal recommendations to take any
nutritional supplements such as herbal supplements, **fish oil,
beneficial bacteria,** or **probiotics.** Several studies are currently
looking at this issue.

The gut is filled with many types of bacteria that assist in
the digestion of food and the production of some vitamins.
During the past decade, interest has grown in the possibility
of stimulating the growth of beneficial gut bacteria as a way
to ward off or treat disease. These bacteria can be augmented
by feeding them nutrients that stimulate their growth or by
supplementing patients with oral bacterial preparations that
colonize the gut. Both approaches are collectively known as
probiotics.

One use for beneficial bacteria may be in food production.
Several studies have considered the possibility of substituting
beneficial bacteria for baker's yeast in fermentation during
wheat-bread production or adding beneficial bacteria later
in the process. The commercially available probiotic product
called **VSL #3,** for example, is a mixture of several strains of

Fish oil

A nutritional supple-
ment with many
health benefits,
including the
ability to suppress
inflammation.

Beneficial bacteria

Bacteria that live
in the intestine,
assist in digestion,
and protect the
body against other
harmful bacteria.

Probiotics

Supplements that
increase the number
of beneficial bacteria
in the intestine.

VSL #3

A commercially
available probiotic
supplement of
beneficial bacteria.

live beneficial bacteria. It has been used in laboratory studies of wheat-based bread production. In the lab, blood taken from patients with CD was processed and exposed to regularly produced bread proteins and to bread dough proteins treated with VSL #3. The VSL #3–treated proteins demonstrated little or no celiac antibody reactivity. The results of this study suggest that using the beneficial bacteria in VSL #3 in the baking process or as an oral supplement might theoretically decrease the immune reaction to gluten.

However, a search of the medical literature did not turn up any completed clinical studies on CD and the use of oral pro-biotics in actual patients. There is an ongoing study of celiac patients in Israel using a probiotic product called Probactrix, which is a strain of *Escherichia coli* (*E. coli*) bacteria that does not cause disease.

Probiotics have been studied clinically both in patients with irritable bowel syndrome and in the laboratory for this indica-tion. Beneficial bacteria, including lactobacilli, bifidobacteria, and VSL #3, have shown an ability to improve IBS symptoms and laboratory measures of IBS. Possible mechanisms of ac-tion are improved digestion of nutrients, decreased inflam-mation, improved immune function, improved gut motility, decreased toxicity of bile, and more colonic fluid absorption. Probiotic bacteria have also been shown in studies to improve gas and bloating in patients.

The use of fish oil or **omega-3 fatty acid** dietary supplements is common. Possible benefits include improved blood lip-ids (cholesterol and triglycerides), decreased inflammation, and decreased risk of heart disease and stroke. Some studies suggest that certain cancer risks are decreased with fish oil supplements or diets high in cold-water fish. In particular, fish oil supplementation has been shown to help in inflam-matory bowel diseases, Crohn's disease, and ulcerative colitis. The hallmark of these diseases is inflammation of the intes-tines, which can be improved, and other anti-inflammatory

Omega-3 fatty acid
A type of oil generally found in fish that decreases inflammation.

medication dosing decreased when patients take omega-3 supplements on a regular basis.

No studies have addressed the role of fish oil supplements in CD, but a small study did examine blood fatty acid profiles in patients with several types of gastrointestinal diseases (including CD). The researchers found abnormal blood fatty acid profiles in patients with sprue—namely, a deficiency of the essential fatty acids. The authors of this study noted that the abnormality may be related to dietary fat absorption and could result in impaired renewal and formation of cells that line the gut. They recommended addition of omega-3 and omega-6 fats to patients' diets to correct these deficits.

The advantages of probiotics and omega-3 (fish oil) fatty acid supplements are intriguing and clearly require more clinical study in patients. There are some suggestions in the existing data that these supplements may benefit patients with gastrointestinal diseases. I do not generally recommend their use for my patients simply because the jury is still out on this issue. Based on the literature, it may be reasonable to try this approach because these supplements are generally safe. The only major downside to their regular use is the cost and the inconvenience of taking several pills per day.

PART SEVEN

Dermatitis Herpetiformis

What is dermatitis herpetiformis?

Are there any other skin diseases associated with celiac disease?

What is the treatment for dermatitis herpetiformis?

More . . .

80. What is dermatitis herpetiformis?

Dermatitis herpetiformis is an intensely itchy, blistering rash that occurs on the elbows, knees, buttocks, trunk, and scalp.

Dermatitis herpetiformis (DH) is an intensely itchy, blistering rash that occurs on the elbows, knees, buttocks, trunk, and scalp. The itchiness can be stressful and maddening, impair sleep, and cause great suffering owing to its unrelenting nature. Blisters are usually tiny (less than 0.25 inch), but are rarely seen in the doctor's office because they are commonly scratched away by the time of the appointment. This makes diagnosis difficult, often delaying it for years and requiring multiple visits to physicians before the appropriate diagnosis is made. The rash of DH is commonly misdiagnosed as eczema, insect bites, contact dermatitis, hives, shingles, herpes, or even a secondary complication of stress.

Dermatitis herpetiformis is fairly rare, with population-based studies demonstrating a rate of 1 to 10 cases per 100,000 people. Like CD, DH runs in families. Approximately 10 to 15 percent of the first-degree relatives of a patient with DH will have CD or DH. As with CD, the family clustering of DH is related to genetic transmission, and the HLA patterns for both CD and DH are similar. Twenty to thirty percent of the general population carries the HLA-DQ2 gene, compared to 90 percent of those individuals with DH. There is also an association between DH and HLA-DQ8, which can occur in the face of HLA-DQ2-negative disease.

The average age of onset for DH is approximately 38 years, somewhat older than the age of onset for CD. Dermatitis herpetiformis can occur in children, and its identification should prompt testing for CD. Unlike CD, which has a female predominance of cases, DH has a slight male predominance; the male-to-female ratio is 1.4–2:1. Dermatitis herpetiformis is also associated with several other autoimmune diseases. For example, one third of patients with DH also have thyroid abnormalities. There is a slight increased risk of lymphoma in DH that is improved with a gluten-free diet.

81. What is the relationship between dermatitis herpetiformis and celiac disease?

Virtually all patients with DH will be shown to have CD by blood testing or small intestinal biopsy. Indeed, some authorities suggest that DH is "CD of the skin." Conversely, only 10 percent of patients with CD also have DH. The severity of inflammation and villus atrophy on intestinal biopsies does not correlate with the severity of skin symptoms. Approximately 20 percent of patients with DH have normal intestinal biopsies, another 20 percent have complete flattening of the villi, and the other 60 percent fall somewhere in between the two extremes.

Clinically, symptoms of DH vary, though 10 to 20 percent of DH patients have classic GI symptoms with malabsorption. Twenty percent of DH patients have atypical symptoms, and 60 percent of patients have asymptomatic CD. The close relationship between CD and DH is partially explained by the common genetic association of HLA-DQ2 and HLA-DQ8, which are present in almost all of these patients. This association also explains the increased family risks and clustering of DH cases within families.

All patients with DH should undergo testing for CD, consisting of blood antibodies and endoscopy with intestinal biopsy. Of course, a diagnosis of DH essentially means you have CD. Small intestinal biopsies are normal in 20 percent of patients with DH. Nevertheless, both DH and CD respond to a gluten-free diet within a few months and recur with resumption of dietary gluten. All patients with DH should be screened for nutrient and vitamin deficiencies as well as thyroid, liver, and bone disease.

Virtually all patients with DH will be shown to have CD by blood testing or small intestinal biopsy. Indeed, some authorities suggest that DH is "CD of the skin."

Dermatitis Herpetiformis

82. Are there any other skin diseases associated with celiac disease?

In addition to DH, several other autoimmune skin diseases are associated with CD (Table 25). Approximately 5 percent of celiac patients experience recurrent bouts of mouth ulcers called aphthous stomatitis. **Psoriasis** is a common autoimmune skin disorder characterized by red, inflamed skin and scaly, thick plaques on the arms, legs, trunk, buttocks, and scalp. Its cause is unknown but this disease frequently occurs in patients with CD and is generally unresponsive to a gluten-free diet.

Eczema is another very common autoimmune skin disorder, affecting 1 in 5 children and 1 in 12 adults. One type of eczema, called atopic eczema, is believed to be a hereditary condition that runs in families. People with atopic eczema are sensitive to allergens in their environment, resulting in an overactive immune response. This response leads to red, irritated skin that can crack and produce local bleeding.

Vitiligo is an autoimmune skin condition affecting 1 to 2 percent of the population that is characterized by white patches of skin. The loss of pigmentation can also affect the hair, resulting in white patches of skin and hair. In this disease, an overactive immune system attacks the skin **melanocytes**, the cells that produce the tan pigment in skin; the outcome of their destruction is areas of skin without pigment.

Alopecia areata is an autoimmune skin condition in which hair follicles are attacked and destroyed, resulting in the patchy

Psoriasis
An inflammatory condition of the skin characterized by thick, scaly plaques.

Vitiligo
An autoimmune skin condition characterized by patchy loss of pigmentation with white spots.

Melanocyte
A cell generally found in the skin that produces pigment.

Alopecia areata
An autoimmune disease characterized by patchy hair loss on the head or body.

Table 25 Skin Diseases Associated with Celiac Disease

Dermatitis herpetiformis
Eczema
Psoriasis
Alopecia areata (baldness or hair loss)
Vitiligo
Aphthous stomatitis (mouth sores or ulcers)

loss of hair on the scalp and body. This problem, which affects 1.7 percent of the U.S. population, can start in childhood and ultimately progress to baldness or total body hair loss.

All of these skin conditions are fairly common in the general population but can be increased in the setting of underlying CD. With the exception of DH, they do not improve upon adoption of a gluten-free diet.

83. How is dermatitis herpetiformis diagnosed?

The diagnosis of DH is based on a history of recurring itchy, blistering rashes on the extensor surfaces of the arms, legs, and trunk with the classic findings seen on skin biopsy. Antibody blood testing for CD with the EMA or tTG test is positive in only 70 percent of patients with DH; thus 30 percent of these individuals are negative for these antibodies. This discrepancy is explained by the fact that the severity of DH does not correlate with the degree of intestinal inflammation and damage seen on small intestine biopsy. By contrast, the presence of celiac antibodies does correlate with the degree of damage in the small intestine. Accordingly, this weaker relationship makes antibody testing less reliable as a means of diagnosing DH.

Like the diagnosis of CD, the diagnosis of DH is not based on symptoms. Instead, the "gold standard" for diagnosing DH is a skin biopsy of normal-appearing skin located immediately next to a blistering lesion. False-negative biopsies are common, as the specimen must be examined appropriately and processed a special way to preserve the signs of DH. In other words, the pathologist examining the biopsy must be aware of the potential for DH and process the specimen with a stain to detect IgA antibodies in the skin. The presence of granular-appearing IgA deposits in the **dermal papillae** (the area under the top layer of skin) confirms the diagnosis of DH.

The "gold standard" for diagnosing DH is a skin biopsy of normal-appearing skin located immediately next to a blistering lesion. The presence of granular-appearing IgA deposits in the dermal papillae confirms the diagnosis.

Dermal papillae

A layer of the skin that is abnormal on a skin biopsy in someone with dermatitis herpetiformis.

Dermatitis Herpetiformis

84. What is the treatment for dermatitis herpetiformis?

The main treatment or "cure" for DH is a gluten-free diet, which will improve the rash and the underlying CD, thereby reducing complications. Dermatitis herpetiformis is very sensitive to gluten ingestion, and a flare-up of DH resulting from ingestion of dietary gluten can take several weeks to resolve.

Several medications are available for DH. These drugs improve the itching but do not treat the underlying immune reaction caused by IgA deposition in the skin. **Dapsone (sulfapyridine)** is an older antibiotic that will improve the itching but has a number of side effects and toxicities. Topical creams that suppress the immune system, such as steroids, **tacrolimus (Protopic),** and **pimecrolimus (Elidel),** may also be effective in relieving symptoms but do not change the underlying pathological process.

The gluten-free diet is the most effective treatment for both stopping the immune process underlying DH and treating coexisting CD. Approximately 80 percent of all DH patients respond to this diet, though dapsone may be needed to control some symptoms.

Dapsone (sulfapyridine)

A drug used to treat the symptoms of dermatitis herpetiformis.

Tacrolimus (Protopic)

An anti-inflammatory medication used to treat some skin conditions.

Pimecrolimus (Elidel)

A medication used to treat inflammatory conditions of the skin.

PART EIGHT

Diseases Associated with Celiac Disease

What is the association between selective IgA deficiency and celiac disease?

What is the association between type 1 diabetes and celiac disease?

What is the association between autoimmune disease and celiac disease?

More...

85. What is the association between selective IgA deficiency and celiac disease?

The immune system protects us from infection, mediates inflammation, and aids in wound healing. One part of the immune system consists of antibodies (immunoglobulins)— proteins produced by white blood cells that bind to other proteins recognized as foreign. For example, when you are vaccinated for hepatitis B, you are inoculated with a protein derived from other proteins found on the surface of this virus. Your body responds by producing antibodies to the hepatitis protein. Then, the next time you are exposed to this virus, the existing antibodies will immediately recognize and bind to it, stimulating other cells to come and destroy the invader.

Many different types of antibodies or immunoglobulins (called IgA, IgD, IgE, IgG, and IgM) are found in the body, each of which performs a different job. Some types travel in the blood to bind foreign proteins (IgG and IgM), others initiate allergic reactions (IgE), and yet another type blocks bacteria or viruses from entering the lining of the gut (IgA). The role of IgA, for example, is to protect the lungs, airways, sinuses, and gut from infection.

There are many defects in the immune system that can predispose a person to developing infection. Some immune defects or deficiencies are present from birth, others are acquired, and still others arise after infection (such as with HIV or AIDS). The spectrum of immune deficiency is quite variable and ranges from mild to severe (for example, leading to death at an early age). The most common defect is selective IgA deficiency, which affects about 1 in 500 people. Selective IgA deficiency usually manifests as recurrent ear and throat infections in children and as sinus infections, bronchitis, and pneumonia in adults. The risk of infection is variable, and some people with selective IgA deficiency have few or no symptoms.

Another problem associated with selective IgA deficiency is increased risk of developing autoimmune disease—in particular, rheumatoid arthritis, lupus, thyroid disease, or idiopathic thrombocytopenia purpura (low platelet count). Allergic diseases such as asthma, eczema, seasonal allergies, and food allergies (including CD) are also more likely when an individual has selective IgA deficiency. Selective IgA deficiency is 10 to 15 times more common in patients with CD than the general population, with 1.7 to 3 percent of celiacs having this disorder. Conversely, 8 percent of all people with selective IgA deficiency also have CD.

As mentioned in Question 38, standard blood testing for CD is based on the presence of IgA antibodies to gliadin (AGA), endomysium (EMA), and tissue transglutaminase (tTG). Because patients with selective IgA deficiency do not make IgA, they will have false-negative blood testing for CD, leading to a missed diagnosis in 1 to 3 of every 100 cases of CD. Alternative testing for CD is available in such circumstances. In fact, the IgG EMA and tTG tests have nearly 100 percent sensitivity in IgA-deficient patients. When screening high-risk patients for CD, only the IgA tests are currently recommended. If these results are negative yet a high suspicion of CD persists, then an IgA level can be done to determine the patient's ability to produce IgA. If the IgA level is very low or absent, then IgG testing can be performed.

86. What is the association between type 1 diabetes and celiac disease?

The association between CD and type 1 diabetes has been well recognized for more than 40 years. Studies of U.S. children and adults with type 1 diabetes have demonstrated that 4 to 6 percent have CD. Both disorders share the same genetic predisposition (that is, the association with HLA-DQ2 and HLA-DQ8). Some evidence suggests that CD can predate diabetes and that a delay in diagnosis of CD during childhood

Because patients with selective IgA deficiency do not make IgA, they will have false-negative blood testing for CD, leading to a missed diagnosis in 1 to 3 of every 100 cases of CD.

Pancreatic islet cells

The cells that make insulin.

may increase a person's risk of developing diabetes. In addition, autoantibodies to **pancreatic islet cells** (which produce insulin) have been discovered in untreated celiacs and disappear with gluten restriction.

Several studies have examined how a gluten-free diet affects celiacs with type 1 diabetes. In these studies, the baseline data on weight, body mass index (BMI), hemoglobin A_{1C} (HbA_{1C}, a marker of elevated blood sugar), and insulin dosing were lower in CD patients compared to patients without this disease. After 12 months on a gluten-free diet, all markers in the patients with CD were the same as those in the normal controls. The same data also demonstrated an improvement in weight loss in underweight patients but no benefit in diabetic blood sugar control or insulin needs with the diet.

In a Hungarian study, researchers screened 205 children with type 1 diabetes for CD and found 24 positive cases. The baseline BMI of these 24 children was low compared to the BMI levels for the children who did not have CD. Body mass index improved when the children followed a gluten-free diet, though their insulin requirements increased and their HbA_{1C} levels did not improve. This Hungarian study confirmed the results previously reported—namely, that the benefit of a gluten-free diet for patients with diabetes is unclear. Nevertheless, the diet does benefit the underlying CD.

Autoimmune disease occurs when the body identifies part of itself as "foreign" and attacks the "invader," resulting in inflammation and damage.

Because of the strong association between type 1 diabetes and CD, screening of diabetics should be considered particularly if they have any GI symptoms.

87. What is the association between autoimmune disease and celiac disease?

Autoimmune disease occurs when the body identifies part of itself as "foreign" and attacks the perceived "invader," resulting in inflammation and damage. In such a case, a defect in the immune system renders it overactive, causing it to target normal proteins and stimulating an immune response. This response includes the production of autoantibodies, or antibodies to normally occurring proteins that are misidentified as bacteria, viruses, or some other "foreign" protein. When an autoantibody binds to a normal protein, it initiates a cascade of inflammation that starts with other cells migrating to the area and continues with the release of other proinflammatory mediators.

Autoimmune disease is fairly common, affecting approximately 5 percent of the general population. Because there is some sort of defect in the immune system, autoimmune diseases tend to occur together. As a consequence, affected individuals frequently have several coexisting autoimmune diseases. Patients with CD, for example, commonly have some other autoimmune process. One study found a significantly higher rate of autoimmune disease in CD patients (14 percent) than in patients without CD (2.8 percent). The risk of developing other autoimmune diseases increased with the duration of gluten exposure, suggesting that early institution of a gluten-free diet may decrease this risk.

The cause of autoimmune disease is unknown, but several factors likely play a role in its development. Genetics and inherited genes clearly influence this process, as the HLA type helps to regulate the immune system. This explains why autoimmune diseases tend to run in families: The genes for HLA type are passed from parent to child. Most patients with CD carry HLA-DQ2, and the remainder carry HLA-DQ8; thus it may be reasonable to assume that these types increase the risk of autoimmunity. This link has been noted for type 1 diabetes, dermatitis herpetiformis (DH), and autoimmune thyroid disease, for example, but it does not explain other autoimmune diseases.

Many associated autoimmune diseases can occur in the setting of CD (Figure 10).

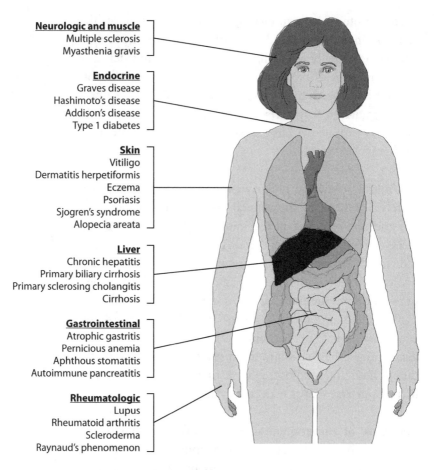

Neurologic and muscle
Multiple sclerosis
Myasthenia gravis

Endocrine
Graves disease
Hashimoto's disease
Addison's disease
Type 1 diabetes

Skin
Vitiligo
Dermatitis herpetiformis
Eczema
Psoriasis
Sjogren's syndrome
Alopecia areata

Liver
Chronic hepatitis
Primary biliary cirrhosis
Primary sclerosing cholangitis
Cirrhosis

Gastrointestinal
Atrophic gastritis
Pernicious anemia
Aphthous stomatitis
Autoimmune pancreatitis

Rheumatologic
Lupus
Rheumatoid arthritis
Scleroderma
Raynaud's phenomenon

Figure 10   Autoimmune diseases associated with celiac disease.

Graves' disease

An autoimmune disease characterized by an overactive thyroid and possible eye changes.

Hashimoto's thyroiditis (Hashimoto's disease)

An autoimmune disease of the thyroid, characterized by possible swelling, pain, and underactivity.

88. What is the association between thyroid disease and celiac disease?

The thyroid is a small gland in the neck that regulates metabolism. In essence, it is the "thermostat" of the body. The thyroid produces thyroid hormone, which regulates body temperature, energy level, gut function, growth, weight, and heart and muscle function. In short, this hormone can affect virtually any organ system. Autoimmune thyroid disease is very common and can lead to an overactive thyroid (hyperthyroidism), called **Graves' disease,** or an underactive thyroid (hypothyroidism), called **Hashimoto's thyroiditis (Hashimoto's disease).**

Symptoms of an overactive thyroid (Graves' disease) include heart palpitations or rapid rate, weight loss, anxiety, sweating, diarrhea, intolerance to hot weather, and poor sleep. A physical sign of Graves' disease is protruding eyes; normally, little or no white part of the eye (the sclera) should be seen over the colored part (the iris), because it should be covered by the eyelid. Another physical sign is an enlarged or swollen thyroid (goiter), which can be tender. Graves' disease is treated with medication that suppresses thyroid hormone production. Frequently, part or all of the thyroid must be destroyed either with surgery or with a radioactive iodine drink that collects in the thyroid gland.

Frequently, an overactive thyroid may be completely destroyed or can "burn out," resulting in hypothyroidism. Symptoms of an underactive thyroid (Hashimoto's disease) include fatigue, depression, weight gain, muscle weakness, constipation, and intolerance to cold weather. Hashimoto's disease is treated with thyroid hormone replacement therapy.

Both Graves' and Hashimoto's diseases are autoimmune diseases in which anti-thyroid antibodies are detectable in the blood. Approximately 10 to 15 percent of patients with CD have autoimmune thyroid disease, and there is an even split between overactive and underactive thyroid disease. Many of these patients are asymptomatic and said to have "subclinical" thyroid disease. Studies of patients with autoimmune thyroid disease who were screened for CD demonstrated an increased rate of CD, ranging from 2 to 4 percent.

Following a gluten-free diet occasionally improves autoimmune thyroid disease in patients with CD, regardless of whether they have symptomatic or subclinical disease. More commonly, compliance with the gluten-free diet means that thyroid hormone replacement therapy can be reduced because drug absorption from the gut improves. The symptoms of CD and thyroid disease—diarrhea, weight loss, fatigue, weakness, and muscle dysfunction—often mimic each other, and with a gluten-free diet both sets of symptoms may improve.

Diseases Associated with Celiac Disease

167

89. What is the association between liver disease and celiac disease?

Celiac disease can be associated with several liver disorders, including hepatitis and abnormal or elevated liver tests.

Celiac disease can be associated with several liver disorders, including hepatitis and abnormal or elevated liver tests. In such cases, the autoimmune nature of CD might be the cause of the liver disease, as many liver diseases have an autoimmune etiology. Celiac disease may also be associated with more severe liver disease. For example, a small European study showed that 4.5 percent of liver transplant patients had CD. Celiac disease increases the risk of liver cancer by 2 to 3 times and the risk of death from cirrhosis of the liver by 7 to 8 times. Elevated liver tests may be the only manifestation of CD in some patients, and these abnormalities can be improved with a gluten-free diet. Approximately 2 to 9 percent of patients with abnormal liver tests have CD.

Patients with primary biliary cirrhosis are 15 times more likely to develop CD than individuals without liver disease. Patients with cryptogenic liver disease have a 15-fold increased risk for positive blood testing for CD compared to members of the general population.

One population-based study from Sweden looked at liver disease in nearly 14,000 patients with CD. The results were actually quite concerning, as shown in Table 26. This table compares patients with diagnosed CD to individuals without CD. The numbers are quoted in terms of relative risk (RR). For example, if RR = 2, then the group is two times as likely to have a disease. Table 26 focuses on patients with CD who were diagnosed with liver disease later in life. It shows, for instance, that patients with CD are 10 times more likely to develop primary biliary cirrhosis than individuals without CD.

Table 27 provides data on individuals with liver disease who were subsequently diagnosed with CD. It shows the relative risk of getting CD if preexisting liver disease is present. Thus Table 27 is the converse of Table 26. For example, it shows that patients with primary biliary cirrhosis are 15 times more likely to develop CD than individuals without liver disease. Overall, prior liver disease was associated with a 4 to 6 times greater risk of developing CD later in life.

Table 26   The Risk of Developing Liver Disease for Patients with Preexisting Celiac Disease

Liver Disease	RR
Acute hepatitis	5.21
Chronic hepatitis	5.84
Primary sclerosing cholangitis	4.46
Fatty liver disease	6.06
Primary biliary cirrhosis	10.16
Liver failure	3.62
Liver cirrhosis	2.23

Table 27   The Risk of Developing Celiac Disease for Patients with Preexisting Liver Disease

Liver Disease	RR of Celiac Disease
Acute hepatitis	4.38
Chronic hepatitis	5.79
Primary sclerosing cholangitis	4.42
Fatty liver disease	5.83
Primary biliary cirrhosis	15.00
Liver failure	8.33
Liver cirrhosis	5.83

Another category not addressed in this study was "cryptogenic" chronic liver disease, or liver disease with an unknown cause. A different study that focused on patients with cryptogenic liver disease showed that these individuals had a 15-fold increased risk for positive blood testing for CD compared to members of the general population.

The "take home message" from these studies is simple: If you have CD, your doctor should periodically check your liver tests to see whether you have developed a liver abnormality. The reverse is also true: Patients with abnormal liver tests should undergo celiac testing. Furthermore, patients with known liver disease—particularly those with an autoimmune disease such as primary biliary cirrhosis or chronic hepatitis—should be checked for CD. Given these data, it may be reasonable to check for CD in all patients with liver disease or abnormal liver tests.

PART NINE

Complications

What are refractory sprue and collagenous sprue?

What is ulcerative jejunitis?

What is the relationship between celiac disease and cancer (including lymphoma)?

More . . .

90. What are refractory sprue and collagenous sprue?

Patients with long-standing CD, even if they follow a strict diet, sometimes redevelop celiac symptoms of diarrhea, weight loss, and malabsorption. Usually, recurrent symptoms come from known or unknown gluten ingestion or some other process such as microscopic colitis or lactose intolerance. Rarely, symptoms are from refractory CD or collagenous sprue, both of which are characterized by severe malabsorption that does not respond to a strict gluten-free diet. Malabsorption is manifested as low blood protein levels, weight loss, and malnutrition with vitamin deficiencies.

Typically, endoscopy and small intestinal biopsy of patients with these conditions will show inflammation with flattening of the villi. In collagenous sprue, patients develop fibrosis—that is, deposits of bands of **collagen** under the villi. Because these complications are not from gluten ingestion, antibody testing for the EMA or tTG should be negative, which can help confirm the diagnosis of refractory CD.

Collagen

The protein in all tissues that holds things together and adds strength to hair, skin, and nails.

Refractory CD tends to occur in older patients or those who carry two copies of the gene for HLA-DQ2. Two types of refractory CD are distinguished: one form that responds to medication and another form that can be a precursor to lymphoma (a cancer affecting the small intestine). By definition, both types do not respond to the gluten-free diet. The second form of refractory disease is covered in detail in Questions 91 and 92, which deal with ulcerative jejunitis and lymphoma, respectively. The treatable version of refractory CD is discussed here.

Total parenteral nutrition (TPN)

Intravenous feeding used when the gut has failed.

Owing to the malabsorption, treatment of refractory CD requires nutrition support and correction of vitamin and mineral deficiencies. Because nutrient absorption is severely impaired, intravenous feeding called **total parenteral nutrition (TPN)** may be required. This kind of liquid nutrition is infused directly into the bloodstream, bypassing the intestines. Total parenteral nutrition can provide calories, protein, vitamins, and minerals and is commonly used to sustain patients with many different kinds of severe gut disease.

The intestinal inflammation of refractory CD is treated with anti-inflammatory medications such as **steroids;** examples include **prednisone** and **budesonide.** Other medications may be required if there is an inadequate response to steroids or if the side effects are unacceptable. For example, **immunosuppressants** or **immunomodulators** may be required. These drugs, which are used to "calm" the immune system, historically have been used in patients who have undergone organ transplants to prevent rejection of the "foreign" organ. Examples include **azathioprine** and **Imuran,** both of which can be prescribed to reduce the dose and decrease the side effects associated with steroids.

Unfortunately, refractory CD does not always respond to medical therapy. This problem can be very difficult to treat, resulting in hospitalization for dehydration, electrolyte abnormalities, and (rarely) death.

91. What is ulcerative jejunitis?

A rare complication of CD in patients with refractory symptoms unresponsive to steroids is ulcerative jejunitis. This condition goes by a number of names, including ulcerative jejunitis, ulcerative jejunoileitis, and ulcerative ileojejunitis. All are the same disease, however.

Patients with ulcerative jejunitis develop multiple benign-appearing ulcers in the jejunum after many years of having CD and complying with the gluten-free diet. There is a slight female predominance in terms of who is affected by this disease, and it usually occurs in people aged 50 to 60 years old. The symptoms of ulcerative jejunitis are similar to those observed with severe CD: diarrhea, weight loss, malabsorption,

Steroids
Medications used to treat inflammation.

Prednisone
A steroid medication used to suppress inflammation.

Budesonide
A type of steroid medication that suppresses the immune system and is used to treat inflammation.

Immuno-suppressant
See *Immuno-modulators.*

Immuno-modulators
Drugs used to treat autoimmune diseases that suppress the immune system.

Azathioprine
A drug that suppresses the immune system and is commonly used to treat autoimmune disease. It is sometimes used for refractory sprue.

Imuran
A drug that suppresses inflammation and the immune system. It is used to treat autoimmune disease. Also known as azathioprine.

Complications

fevers, and abdominal pain. A narrowing of the small intestines (strictures) may also cause bowel obstructions. Ulcerative jejunitis responds poorly to the gluten-free diet and medications. The prognosis with this disease is poor, with as many as one third of patients dying from this complication.

The major concern with ulcerative jejunitis is the development of small intestinal lymphoma. Lymphoma is a cancer affecting the lymph nodes—and there are a lot of lymph nodes in the intestine. Many authorities on this subject consider ulcerative jejunitis and lymphoma a spectrum of the same disease (with lymphoma being found at the more severe end of the disease spectrum) and suggest that ulcerative jejunitis leads to lymphoma.

The diagnosis of ulcerative jejunitis is difficult to make. Generally, endoscopy with biopsy, CT scan, and other imaging may not help make this diagnosis. Many patients require an operation to examine the intestines and get a full-thickness biopsy—that is, the surgeon cuts a wedge of tissue out of the small intestine and then sews up the opening. Later, the tissue can be examined by a pathologist to determine whether the abnormal inflammation is CD, ulcerative jejunitis, or lymphoma. Special studies can tell whether the inflammatory cells are different cells or many copies of the same cell (lymphoma).

Refractory CD, ulcerative jejunitis, and small intestinal lymphoma should definitely be treated by a gastrointestinal specialist. In such cases, I would recommend referral to a major or teaching hospital.

92. What is the relationship between celiac disease and cancer (including lymphoma)?

The relationship between CD and cancer is well established and has been described in the medical literature for years. There is a well-known association between CD and cancer of the head and neck, esophagus, **adenocarcinoma** of the small intestine, and lymphoma. Many types of lymphoma are related to abnormal cell types; the version seen in conjunction with CD is called enteropathy-associated T-cell lymphoma (EATL).

Enteropathy-associated T-cell lymphoma generally occurs in adults (approximately 60 years old); it does not affect children. If a person has CD, the development of lymphoma may occur over a span as short as five years—but can also take decades. When lymphoma occurs in an individual with CD, the patient has typically been on a gluten-free diet for years and gets new symptoms. These symptoms may include weight loss, diarrhea, pain, fevers, and soaking sweats at night; in addition, a mass can sometimes be felt on exam of the abdomen. There can be bleeding, bowel obstruction, and **perforation,** which can require surgery in as many as 50 percent of patients. The cancer can involve the small intestine, lymph nodes of the abdomen, stomach, colon, liver, and spleen.

Evaluation for lymphoma should be performed for patients with CD who have refractory symptoms that do not respond to a gluten-free diet. Testing may include a CT scan, barium x-rays, endoscopy, and colonoscopy. The final diagnosis requires examination of a small intestine tissue sample obtained at endoscopy or a full-thickness biopsy from surgery.

Treatment for EATL consists of surgery if the disease is localized to one area. This is rarely the case, however. Chemotherapy may help when the cancer is more widespread. Unfortunately, the outlook for patients with EATL is poor. For example, a recent study from the United Kingdom found that 13 percent of patients were alive 2.5 years after their diagnosis with this disease.

Thankfully, EATL is rare, though it does account for 35 percent of all small bowel lymphomas. In Western population studies, EATL has been found at a rate of 0.5 to 1 case per

Adenocarcinoma

A type of cancer that on microscopic exam forms glands. Examples include prostate, stomach, pancreas, colon, some lung, and esophageal cancers.

Perforation

A hole in the wall of the intestine that requires surgery to repair.

Complications

1 million people. To put this rate in perspective, 1 in every 11 women gets breast cancer and 1 in every 20 people gets colon cancer. Thus the overall risk of EATL is low, but CD clearly increases your risk of developing lymphoma. When a large U.K. study followed a population of patients with CD for 5684 person-years, researchers found that the overall lymphoma risk was increased 5-fold and the small bowel lymphoma risk was increased 40-fold. This risk sounds high but should be looked at this way: There were 4 cases of lymphoma and 1 case of EATL in this study in more than 5500 person-years. Several studies suggest that a gluten-free diet may reduce this risk.

93. Is there an increased risk of mortality in celiac disease?

Another way to ask this question is, "Is there an excess risk of death from CD?" Several studies have looked into this issue and found that mortality (the death rate) is increased 1.9- to 3.4-fold in the setting of CD. Careful analysis shows that the increased death rate applied to those patients who were symptomatic, had malabsorption, had a prolonged delay in diagnosis, or did not adhere to a strict gluten-free diet. No excess death rate was seen in patients with mild or asymptomatic CD. The increased number of deaths seen in patients with CD was related predominantly to cancer, including EATL (see Question 92), other lymphomas, and cancer of the esophagus, stomach, pancreas, bile ducts, small bowel, lungs, thyroid, skin, and blood (leukemia). Other sources of the increased death rate included malabsorption with refractory CD and ulcerative jejunitis.

94. Does a gluten-free diet prevent complications of celiac disease?

A gluten-free diet improves the symptoms associated with CD and DH, malabsorption, and vitamin deficiencies. Several studies have shown that the risk of developing cancer for patients with CD is reduced with a strict diet. One study reported the risk of lymphoma was reduced by 60 percent with such a diet. Another study of patients with DH demonstrated that those who developed cancer were less likely to be faithful to the diet in terms of gluten avoidance. Other studies have reported that patients on a strict diet had no increased cancer risk. A large Swedish study looked at the age of diagnosis of CD and cancer risk, concluding that children who were diagnosed by age 10 had no increased cancer risk when they followed a strict diet.

Because of the increased cancer risk observed in CD, I always recommend strict adherence to a gluten-free diet to my patients. This is the only way to minimize your overall cancer risk and chance of getting a rare but aggressive cancer. In addition, the benefits of a gluten-free diet for patients with CD and DH include improvements in symptoms and decreased risk of other associated conditions such as anemia, osteoporosis, and malabsorption. Body composition is also improved, with increased muscle and bone mass being noted in patients who follow a gluten-free diet.

95. Is obesity common in treated celiac disease?

Historically, CD has been characterized by weight loss, malabsorption, and being underweight. Two thirds (65 percent) of the U.S. population are overweight, and one third are obese (roughly 30 pounds overweight). Studies on adults show that most patients diagnosed with CD are either of normal weight or overweight before a gluten-free diet is even started. One study followed 371 patients with CD by examining their baseline weight and subsequent weight changes over two years on a gluten-free diet. At baseline, 5 percent were underweight and 40 percent were overweight or obese. During the two years they followed a gluten-free diet, 80 percent of patients gained weight and 51 percent became overweight or obese.

Complications

There may be several reasons for the weight gain associated with a gluten-free diet. Patients with bloating, diarrhea, and stomach cramps may limit the amount they eat because they are not hungry or find that limiting food helps with their symptoms. They may also restrict their consumption of certain foods, such as dairy or fatty foods, thereby decreasing the total calories eaten. In addition, their doctors may have recommended avoiding certain high-calorie foods to help with symptoms.

Malabsorption is an integral part of CD. In this disease, not only is absorption of vitamins and minerals impaired, but other nutrients, such as dietary fat, are affected as well. In CD, fat—which is difficult to digest and absorb even in normal individuals—is excreted in the stool. Studies on patients with CD have found that they may malabsorb 5 to 15 percent of their total daily calories. In effect, these patients are on a calorie-restricted diet: If they eat 2000 calories per day, they actually absorb only 1700 to 1900 calories. After a gluten-free diet is implemented, however, the CD-associated gut inflammation heals and absorption becomes normal. The 2000 calories eaten is then completely absorbed. Thus the daily number of consumed calories is the same, but the net result is getting 100 to 300 more calories per day. This really adds up, as 1 pound of fat equals 3500 calories. In fact, switching to a gluten-free diet can result in gaining 1 to 3 pounds per month if you do not change your total intake of calories.

This weight gain is further compounded by the improved sense of well-being on a gluten-free diet if the person has been ill for many years. Once you feel better, the tendency is to eat more.

Finally, gluten-containing foods contain high amounts of carbohydrates, which are actually a good source of nutrition. A balanced diet high in carbohydrates helps to maintain your weight by limiting your total fat intake to 30 percent or less of daily calories. With a gluten-free diet, intake of carbohydrates is reduced and fats tend to substitute for them. These fatty foods are more calorically dense, meaning more calories per serving and leading to increased total calories eaten.

All of these issues contribute to the weight gain commonly associated with switching to a gluten-free diet. Follow-up appointments with a dietitian are very important for management of a balanced gluten-free diet, avoidance of excessive weight gain, and maintenance of an appropriate, healthy weight.

Complications

PART TEN

Patient Resources

Are there support groups for celiac disease?

Where can I get more information on the gluten-free diet?

What support or information is available for children with celiac disease?

More . . .

96. Are there support groups for celiac disease?

Support groups and patient advocacy groups are extremely helpful to individuals with CD. Celiac disease is a common disorder, affecting about 1 in 100 Americans, or nearly 3 million people. Gluten is everywhere and very difficult to avoid. It is an unlabeled contaminant in beauty products, a component in some stationery products, and a binder in some drugs. Gluten is also difficult to avoid when dining out. I very strongly recommend that patients with CD join a support group to help them cope with the challenges of living a gluten-free life. Participation in such a group can range from online activities, such as receiving newsletters and other communications, to joining local groups.

The only way to avoid gluten is through knowledge and education—which is the reason why I wrote this book. All patients with newly diagnosed CD need education on their disease, including information on which ingredients and foods may be a source of potential illness. This is a very difficult process because the gluten-free diet is very restrictive and limited, and life is full of temptations. With time and improved health from the gluten-free diet, however, this process reinforces itself and diminishes the tendency to cheat. Talking about problematic issues like these can be extremely helpful for patients with the same disease, and support groups can provide this forum.

You do not have to go it alone. The information on a gluten-free diet already exists—you just have to find it.

The educational part of the gluten-free diet is learning which foods, supermarkets, and restaurants are safe. Happily, education regarding a gluten-free diet is widely available. You do not have to go it alone. The information already exists—you just have to find it. Reading books like this one is helpful as a resource, but I encourage you to go further by investigating some of the weblinks I have provided. Joining a support group is a terrific resource for obtaining gluten-free information and learning which food items or brands of foods are safe. Some groups have regular meetings and invite speakers to discuss various issues related to CD.

Support groups also perform an important role by promoting disease advocacy. Given that 3 million people in the United States have CD, they collectively have the strength to educate others about CD and the gluten-free diet. They may be able to persuade food manufacturers to label products more effectively, stating that they are gluten-free, or even bring new gluten-free products to market. Talking with restaurant leaders can prompt them to create gluten-free menus. Asking supermarkets to provide more gluten-free products, at a reasonable cost, may bring wider choices. Support groups can also promote medical research into a particular disease and help with funding of that research. For these reasons,

Table 28   Celiac Patient Support Groups

Bay Area Celiacs	www.bayareaceliacs.org/support_groups.htm
Canadian Celiac Association	www.celiac.edmonton.ab.ca
Celiac Disease Foundation	www.celiac.org
Celiac Disease On-line Support	www.geocities.com/HotSprings/Spa/4003/delphi.html
Celiac Sprue Association	www.csaceliacs.org
Celiac Support Groups in the U.S. (Great link to local groups by state)	www.enabling.org/ia/celiac/groups/groupsus.html
Cincinnati Celiac Support Group	www.cinciceliac.com
Gluten Free in WNY (Upstate NY)	www.buffaloceliacs.org
Gluten Intolerance Group	www.gluten.net/celiac.html
Healthy Villi (Boston area)	www.healthyvilli.com
National Foundation for Celiac Awareness	www.celiaccentral.org/Links/Support_Groups/54
Rochester Celiac Support (NY)	www.rochesterceliacs.org
Witchita Celiac Support Group	www.geocities.com/glutenfreeceliac

Patient Resources

I always recommend support groups for any patient with a chronic disease.

This is a limited list, particularly for local organizations. Please look at "Celiac Support Groups in the U.S." for a listing by state for your local groups.

Marye comments:

There are a variety of support groups for celiac patients. Call your local health food stores, hospital, and board of health to ask if they are aware of any local support groups. It is also helpful to check the Internet.

97. Where can I get more information on the gluten-free diet?

The first step toward beginning a gluten-free diet is a consultation with a dietitian. These healthcare professionals are specially trained in designing diets and following patients who require special diets. Dietitians can help people either gain or lose weight; they can also plan a diet with restrictions (such as a gluten-free diet). As part of their job, they can provide you with lists of foods and grains to avoid and indicate which foods are safe to eat. Dietitians can be extremely helpful after you have started a gluten-free diet for follow-up—that is, assessing how things are going. They may also be helpful for celiac patients who continue to have symptoms despite switching to a gluten-free diet and can assist them in determining whether gluten is unknowingly being consumed.

Not all dietitians have the same training, however, and many have specialty interests. If you go to a dietitian for a gluten-free diet but the dietitian specializes in teaching patients with diabetes about a low-sugar diet, for example, he or she may not have the necessary information or may not be up-to-date on the gluten-free diet. If you have met with a dietitian and do not feel like the education was sufficient, various options are open to you. First, talk to your doctor and find out whether there may be a more appropriate dietitian whom you can consult. If this effort fails or there are no other "local" dietitian resources, then you may have to go elsewhere. Many large teaching or specialty hospitals have dietitians who specialize in CD. The hospital where I work has terrific dietitians, but sometimes patients continue to get gluten into their diets. In such cases, I may refer patients to a specially trained celiac dietitian who treats only patients with CD. Your gastroenterologist may be able to help you with this or, alternatively, your dietitian may know where to go.

As mentioned in Question 96, local support groups are a tremendous resource for individuals with CD. Their members may know about dietitians who can help you if you are struggling with the gluten-free diet. A support group may also be able to provide extensive information about which foods, cooking materials, brands, medications, markets, cosmetics, and restaurants may be safe or cater to patients with CD.

Table 29   Online Resources for the Gluten-Free Diet

The "Gluten-free diet guide for families" is a terrific download with many good links	www.celiachealth.org/pdf/ GlutenFreeDietGuideWeb.pdf
The Canadian Celiac Association has a good explanation of the gluten-free diet	www.celiac.ca/EnglishCCA/ egfdiet.html#desc
"Gluten-Free Diet" is a great book I recommend, by expert dietitian Shelley Case	www.glutenfreediet.ca
Celiac Sprue Association has good explanation and resources for the gluten-free diet	www.csaceliacs.org/index.php
Gluten-Free Mall is a shopping site that sells gluten-free products	www.celiac.com/catalog

Many books are available online or at your local bookstore that identify gluten-free foods and brands. Gluten-free cookbooks and restaurant guides for patients with food allergies are also available. Many large markets have a gluten-free section, and your local support group may have recommendations about where to shop. The Internet is a great resource for purchasing products or books and downloading dietary information. Table 29 provides some recommendations of dietary sites, books, and online retailers that sell gluten-free products.

Marye comments:

You can obtain information on the gluten-free diet from the Internet, your local library, the magazine Gluten-Free Living, and many health food stores.

98. What support or information is available for children with celiac disease?

Having a child with CD presents issues and problems for both the parents and the child. Parental issues include the need to understand the disease and the difficulty with enforcing a restrictive diet with a child who may already be a fussy eater. Childhood issues include trying to understand why the child is different and why a gluten-free diet is required.

As with adult CD, there is a lot of information available for parents and children with CD as well as a variety of support groups. Check with your pediatrician or local children's hospital regarding any local resources that may be appropriate for your child. Many books are directed to either parents or children with CD, and recommendations can be found online at major retailers such as Amazon.com or through children's celiac support group websites. Table 30 provides a limited list of children's resources. The link to "Celiac Support Groups in the U.S." will turn up a terrific listing of celiac resources by state and includes pediatric information; it is a great way to start your search.

Table 30 Online Celiac Resources for Families and Children

Celiac Disease Support Group at Children's Hospital Boston	www.childrenshospital.org/clinicalservices/Site2166/mainpageS2166P0.html
Celiac.com has a book R.O.C.K. (raising our celiac kids)	www.celiac.com/st_main.html?p_catid=8
Celiac website for children	http://kidshealth.org/kid/health_problems/stomach/celiac.html
Celiac Disease Foundation	www.celiac.org
Celiac Support Groups in the U.S. (Great link to local groups by state)	www.enabling.org/ia/celiac/groups/groupsus.html
Cincinnati ROCK	www.rock.cinciceliac.com
National Foundation for Celiac Awareness kids corner	www.celiaccentral.org/Kids_Corner/17
NASPGHAN provides a great download for families	www.naspghan.org/assets/diseaseInfo/pdf/GlutenFreeDietGuide-E.pdf

Marye comments:

Many different supermarkets and health food stores have special sections devoted to children [with CD] and foods that they would enjoy. I purchase a lot of the children's special cereal and cookies because of the interesting way the products are packaged. Plus they are delicious!

99. Where can I get more medical information on celiac disease?

There are many sources of medical information on CD. The purpose of this book is simply to provide a comprehensive overview of CD, DH, and the gluten-free diet. I am a doctor, so my job here is to provide the most complete and up-to-date information available and to present it in a patient-friendly way. Because of my bias, this book leans toward the medical issues in CD, including a discussion of dietary factors. My hope is that this book provides most, if not all, of the medical information that a patient with CD needs, and answers your questions. Some medical information on CD found in other sources is specifically geared toward patients; other information is highly technical, being written for healthcare providers. There is also misinformation out there: The Internet is at your fingertips, but it is unfiltered information and you need to do your homework. Make sure that the information comes from a reputable source such as a doctor, dietitian, or major institution before you accept it whole-heartedly.

Table 31   Online Celiac Resources for Medical Information

National Digestive Disease Clearing House, a great overview of CD and download	http://digestive.niddk.nih.gov/ddiseases/pubs/celiac/index.htm http://digestive.niddk.nih.gov/ddiseases/pubs/celiac/celiac.pdf
National Institute of Health links on CD	www.nlm.nih.gov/medlineplus/celiacdisease.html
Mayo Clinic patient information	www.mayoclinic.com/health/celiac-disease/DS00319
American College of Gastroenterology patient information on CD	www.gi.org/patients/gihealth/celiac.asp
MedicineNet.com	www.medicinenet.com/celiac_disease/article.htm

The American Gastroenterological Association's technical review of the diagnosis and management of celiac disease (*Gastroenterology*, 2006, pp. 1981–2002) is a great reference for healthcare providers. It was also a tremendous asset to me in writing this book.

Numerous other books available from medical authorities can provide further information. Do not hesitate to ask your doctor or see a specialist to obtain more information about CD or your specific medical issues. Support groups also provide medical information and may give you an opportunity to discuss medical issues with visiting speakers at local meetings.

PART ELEVEN

Conclusion

What is the future of celiac disease?
Will there be a medication that can treat
this disease?

More . . .

100. What is the future of celiac disease? Will there be a medication that can treat this disease?

While doing the research in preparation for writing this book, I learned a tremendous amount about CD and future directions in its treatment. Clearly, there are many areas in which further medical research is warranted. Following are some of the issues that are targets for investigation:

- What are the causes of gluten allergy?
- Why do certain people who carry the genes for HLA-DQ2 and HLA-DQ8 develop CD, whereas many others do not?
- What is the trigger for CD? Early gluten exposure as an infant? An infection that may fool and turn on the immune system?
- Why do some people manifest CD as young children, whereas others get their first symptoms later in life?
- Do people with latent or potential CD benefit from following a gluten-free diet?
- What is the link between CD, DH, and cancer?
- What is the trigger for autoimmune disease, and what is the relationship between other types of autoimmune disease and CD?
- What is the natural history of the various types of CD, particularly in asymptomatic patients?
- Why is CD so prevalent in certain ethnic groups?
- What about gluten-containing grains; can they be engineered to remove the gluten?

For many diseases that affect humans, scientists have developed animal models that allow them to study the mechanism of disease in depth and try out various treatment options. Currently, no such animal model for CD exists, but one's development would certainly facilitate ongoing research. A model might help researchers find potential cures, treatments, and/or medications to relieve symptoms. It might enable researchers to create better tests for diagnosis of CD, thereby improving the rate of diagnosis and decreasing the number of false-negative and false-positive tests. Improved testing may also be less invasive than the endoscopic examination and biopsy required to confirm CD at present.

Increased education of healthcare professionals regarding CD is required and is occurring slowly. Better education will help more patients with minor or atypical symptoms receive the appropriate diagnosis more quickly. It will also help clinicians understand the relationships among autoimmune diseases, CD, and DH; heighten their awareness of these diseases; and prompt them to pursue testing for CD more aggressively. Indeed, the increased awareness has already led to more testing and the revelation that nearly 1 in 100 Americans has CD. Increased understanding will also shorten the typical delay in making the diagnosis of CD, which has historically been about eight years.

The research into potential medications for CD is intriguing. Currently, enzyme supplements are available for patients with diseases of the pancreas to aid digestion of food. Enzyme supplements are also available for lactose-intolerant individuals to help them digest the offending sugar. Both of these supplements are pills that are taken at the time of eating and enable patients to digest the nutrient that they have lost the ability to digest. The preliminary study of gluten-digesting enzymes (see Question 57) suggests that this approach might potentially be used in the future for patients with CD. The combination enzyme cocktail of EP-B2 and PEP and the ability to digest gluten in a simulated human model represent major steps in this regard.

Other treatment avenues are equally interesting but take a different tack, addressing the mechanism of disease. For example, potential therapies might address the interaction of gluten and the immune system or activation of the inflammatory response. Other therapies might focus on CD-associated

Conclusion

inflammation and its effect on the intestine. Question 57 covered the possibility that this inflammation might result in a leaky gut, as well as the role played by zonulin (and its blocking drug AT-1001) in CD. We are just now beginning to see drug development for CD, and we hope to see even more drug prospects emerge in the future.

Nearly 3 million Americans have CD. As a patient, you have a voice. The motto of the Celiac Sprue Association is "Celiacs helping celiacs." You are workers and consumers and have strength through support groups and economic power. This strength enables you to educate others about CD, including healthcare providers, other patients with newly diagnosed CD, and product manufacturers. It facilitates law makers and the FDA to mandate that gluten content appear on the labeling on products. It makes supermarkets want to cater to customers with food allergies or sensitivities. It encourages food manufacturers to offer more prepared products for those with dietary restrictions. It stimulates drug companies to investigate new potential therapies to satisfy an as-yet-unmet need. Your voice keeps the issues active and in the public eye, allowing progress on many fronts.

Appendix

Recommended Books for More Information

A variety of books on celiac disease are available, including recipe and cookbooks, medical books, and books on the gluten-free diet. Only a short list appears. I urge you to check online (the website of a large bookseller, for instance) to see the many books available.

Case S. *Gluten-Free Diet: A Comprehensive Resource Guide.* Regina, Saskatchewan: Case Nutrition Consulting, 2001.

Celiac Sprue Association. *CSA Product Listing,* 11th edition. Omaha, NE: CSA, 2006.

Green PHR, Jones R. *Celiac Disease:. A Hidden Epidemic.* New York: Harper Collins, 2006.

Lowell JP. *The Gluten-Free Bible.* New York: Henry Holt, 2005.

Resources Used in Writing This Book

In writing this book, my goal was to provide the most up-to-date information possible. The Internet was an invaluable source of information for medical articles and virtually any aspect of celiac disease and diet. Any question regarding celiac disease was answered promptly with the appropriate Google search. The links I provide in this book are all good sources of information. This list is limited, however, and does not include the many medical articles that are cited in this book.

American Gastroenterological Association (AGA) Institute Technical Review on the Diagnosis and Management of Celiac Disease. *Gastroenterology* 131:1981–2002; 2006.
   A recent position paper from the AGA with a great review of celiac disease.

Celiac Disease: Proceedings of the NIH Consensus Conference on Celiac Disease, June 28–30, 2004, Bethesda, MD. *Gastroenterology* 128(suppl 1):4; 2005.
A terrific medical resource featuring several timely medical articles on issues in celiac disease, dermatitis herpetiformis, and the gluten-free diet.

Celiac Sprue Association. *CSA Product Listing,* 11th edition. Omaha, NE: CSA, 2006.
I cannot praise this book enough! All celiac patients should own this dictionary on everything gluten-free.

Parrish CR (Ed). The Celiac Diet: A Series. *Practical Gastroenterology* 30:9–19; 2006.
A series of review articles for healthcare practitioners on dietary issues and celiac disease.

UpToDate. www.uptodate.com. Search for "celiac disease."
UpToDate is on online "textbook" that covers almost all areas of medicine. It includes several state-of-the-art sections on celiac disease in adults and children.

Glossary

A

Absorption: The ability to move nutrients in the intestinal contents through the gut lining and into the bloodstream.

Adenocarcinoma: A type of cancer that on microscopic exam forms glands. Examples include prostate, stomach, pancreas, colon, some lung, and esophageal cancers.

Albumin: A protein produced by the liver that circulates in the blood and is a marker of nutritional status.

Alopecia areata: An autoimmune disease characterized by patchy hair loss on the head or body.

Amaranth: A gluten-free starch.

Ambulatory endoscopy center: A free-standing medical procedure center where endoscopy and colonoscopy are done.

Amenorrhea: The lack of menstrual period for women.

Amino acids: The building blocks for proteins. Dietary proteins are broken down into amino acids during the digestion process to allow for their absorption.

Anaphylaxis: A severe, life-threatening allergic reaction that can be fatal.

Anemia: A low blood cell count or level, which has many causes.

Antiendomysial antibody (EMA): A sensitive blood test commonly used to test for celiac disease. The EMA is an IgA antibody test.

Antigliadin antibody (AGA): An IgA antibody blood test that is fairly sensitive for detection of celiac disease. It can also produce false positive and negative results.

Antispasmodic drugs: A class of medications used to relax the intestines. These drugs are commonly prescribed for patients with irritable bowel syndrome. Examples include Bentyl, Levsin, and Donnatal.

Aphthous mouth ulcers: Recurrent sores or ulcers in the mouth that may be associated with celiac disease.

Aphthous stomatitis: See Aphthous mouth ulcers.

Arrowroot: A gluten-free starch.

AT-1001: An investigational drug, not yet approved by the U.S. Food and Drug Administration that is being studied for celiac disease. It blocks zonulin, keeping the gut from becoming leaky in the setting of inflammation.

Ataxia: Difficulty walking, characterized by a staggering gait.

Atypical celiac disease: Celiac disease that manifests without typical symptoms.

Autism: A disorder beginning at an early age that is characterized by delays or difficulty with communication, language, and social interaction.

Autoimmune disease: A type of disease in which the body attacks itself, causing damage. Examples include vitiligo, rheumatoid arthritis, lupus, and autoimmune hepatitis.

Autoimmune hepatitis (AIH): A chronic, progressive inflammatory disease of the liver in which the body attacks itself. It can result in cirrhosis.

Autoimmune liver disease: See Autoimmune hepatitis.

Azathioprine: A drug that suppresses the immune system and is commonly used to treat autoimmune disease. It is sometimes used for refractory sprue.

B

Bacterial overgrowth: The normal small intestine contains small numbers of bacteria that aid in digestion and make vitamins. In bacterial overgrowth, the number and type of bacteria increase, resulting in diarrhea, weight loss, and vitamin deficiencies.

Barium study: An x-ray examination of the small intestine.

Barley: A gluten-containing grain.

Barley extract (barley malt): A gluten-containing food additive

Beneficial bacteria: Bacteria that live in the intestine, assist in digestion, and protect the body against other harmful bacteria.

Bile: A green liquid made by the liver and stored in the gallbladder that helps to digest fats.

Bile salt diarrhea: A chronic diarrheal illness caused by poor absorption of bile. It is typically treated with cholestyramine.

Biopsy: A procedure in which the physician takes a small piece of tissue from the body for later examination under the microscope.

Bisphosphonates: A class of drugs that is used to treat osteoporosis.

Body mass index (BMI): A measure of weight as a function of height. A BMI of less than 18 is considered underweight, 20 to 25 is normal, 25 to 30 is overweight, and greater than 30 is obese.

Bone density scan: An x-ray test used to measure the mineral content of bone and diagnose osteoporosis and the risk of fracture.

Bone mineral density (BMD): A measure of the mineral content (a marker for osteoporosis).

Bowel obstruction: Blockage of the bowel. It is typically accompanied by symptoms of gas, distention, nausea, and vomiting, and usually requires hospitalization.

Buckwheat: A gluten-free grain.

Budesonide: A type of steroid medication that suppresses the immune system and is used to treat inflammation.

Bulgur: A type of wheat that contains gluten.

C

Capsule endoscope: A pill that is an endoscope.

Carotene: A form of vitamin A that aids healthy vision.

Casein-free diet: Casein is a protein derived from milk. A casein-free and gluten-free diet is sometimes suggested for patients with autism.

Celiac disease (CD): Same as sprue or celiac sprue and gluten-sensitive enteropathy. A food allergy to gluten, which is a protein found in the grains wheat, barley, rye, and possibly oats. An autoimmune disease characterized by inflammation and damage to the small intestine, with resulting malabsorption of nutrients.

Celiac sprue: Another term for celiac disease, sprue, or gluten-sensitive enteropathy.

Cellular immune system: One of the two major parts of the immune system, along with the humoral immune system. The cellular immune system is where various immune cells locate, attract, and destroy bacteria or viruses.

Chickpea: A gluten-free bean used as a starch.

Cirrhosis: An advanced form of liver disease characterized by scarring of the liver and an increased risk of liver failure, cancer, and death.

Citrucil: A synthetic fiber supplement that is available over the counter.

Classic celiac disease: Celiac disease that presents with symptoms of diarrhea, weight loss, and bloating.

Clopidogrel (Plavix): A drug used to thin the blood, thereby preventing heart attack and stroke.

Collagen: The protein in all tissues that holds things together and adds strength to hair, skin, and nails.

Collagenous sprue: A type of difficult or refractory sprue that may require additional medication to suppress the immune system.

Colon: The large intestine, which functions to process and store wastes.

Complete blood count (CBC): A type of blood test that gives information on anemia, infection, and the body's ability to stop bleeding. Measurements of hemoglobin (Hg) and hematocrit (HCT) are part of a CBC.

Corn: A gluten-free source of carbohydrate.

Couscous: A gluten-containing grain.

C-reactive protein (CRP): A very sensitive blood test used to measure the amount of inflammation.

Crohn's disease: An autoimmune inflammatory disease that can affect any part of the gastrointestinal tract. Crohn's disease of the small intestine can mimic celiac disease.

D

Dapsone (sulfapyridine): A drug used to treat the symptoms of dermatitis herpetiformis.

Dental enamel: The white hard covering on teeth. Abnormal dental enamel in children can be a sign of celiac disease.

Dermal papillae: A layer of the skin that is abnormal on a skin biopsy in someone with dermatitis herpetiformis.

Dermatitis herpetiformis (DH): An intensely itchy rash with tiny blisters that occurs on the elbows, wrists, shoulders, and back. Virtually all patients with DH have celiac disease and should go on a gluten-free diet.

DEXA scan: A test that measures bone mineral content, risk of fracture, and osteoporosis.

Digestion: The process of breaking food down into simple sugars, triglycerides, and amino acids. Digestion occurs prior to absorption.

Dinkle: A gluten-containing type of wheat.

Down syndrome: A syndrome of mental retardation that is present at birth. There is a very strong association between Down syndrome and celiac disease. Also called trisomy 21.

Dry beri beri: A vitamin deficiency of thiamine characterized by neurologic symptoms

Duodenum: The first part of the small intestine.

Durum: A gluten-containing type of wheat.

E

Eczema: A scaly, itchy red rash that is associated with autoimmune disease.

Einkorn: A gluten-containing grain.

Emmer: A gluten-containing grain.

Encephalopathy: Mental confusion.

Endocrinologist: A doctor who specializes in the treatment of glandular disorders such as diabetes, thyroid disease, and osteoporosis.

Endoscopy: A medical procedure in which the patient swallows a scope, allowing for examination of the gut and the opportunity to take biopsies.

Enteropathy-associated T-cell lymphoma (EATL): A type of T-cell lymphoma of the small intestine that can, on rare occasions, be a complication of celiac disease.

Enzymes: Proteins produced in the pancreas that break down food to its simplest type of nutrient for subsequent absorption.

EP-B2: An enzyme that digests gluten. It is currently being studied as a treatment for celiac disease.

F

Farina: A gluten-containing type of grain.

Faro: A gluten-containing type of grain.

Fat-soluble vitamin: A vitamin that is absorbed with fat. Fat-soluble vitamins include vitamins A, D, E, and K.

Fatty liver disease: An inflammatory disease of the liver caused by excessive deposits of fat in the liver.

Fava: A gluten-free bean and source of starch.

Fermentum: The material added to grape juice to make religious consecrated wine. It may contain gluten.

Ferritin: The storage form of iron in the body. Also, the blood test used to check for iron deficiency.

First-degree relative: A very closely related family member, such as a parent, a child, or a sibling.

Fish oil: A nutritional supplement with many health benefits, including the ability to suppress inflammation.

Flax: A gluten-free grain.

Flu shot: An annual vaccination against the flu. It is generally recommended for chronically ill individuals, people older than age 65, and small children.

Folic acid (folate): An essential vitamin that can be deficient in malabsorption.

G

Gastroenterologist: A doctor who specializes in treating diseases of the intestine, stomach, esophagus, liver, and pancreas and who does endoscopic procedures related to these organs.

Gene: The groups of DNA that are passed from parent to child that determine various body characteristics like eye and hair color.

Genetic disorder: A disorder or disease passed from parent to child through the genes.

Giardia: A parasite that is usually acquired from contaminated water and that infects the intestine, where it causes symptoms similar to those seen with celiac disease (diarrhea, weight loss, and bloating).

Gluten: A protein found in wheat, rye, and barley that makes dough sticky and gooey.

Gluten free: A food that does not contain any gluten.

Gluten-free diet: A diet completely free of any gluten.

Gluten-sensitive enteropathy: Another name for celiac disease.

Gluten sensitivity: A food sensitivity to gluten that causes symptoms but is not an allergy. In such a patient, testing will be negative for celiac disease.

Glycolax: A type of laxative that is commonly used as preparation for a colonoscopy.

Graham flour: A gluten-containing flour.

Graves' disease: An autoimmune disease characterized by an overactive thyroid and possible eye changes.

H

Hashimoto's thyroiditis (Hashimoto's disease): An autoimmune disease of the thyroid, characterized by possible swelling, pain, and underactivity.

Hematocrit (HCT): A blood test for anemia.

Hemoglobin (Hb): A blood test for anemia.

Hepatitis: An inflammatory condition of the liver that can be chronic, resulting in scarring (cirrhosis) and jaundice.

HLA-DQ2/HLA-DQ8: The two genes that predispose a person to having celiac disease.

Host: The wheat-containing wafer taken at communion to symbolize Christ.

Human immunodeficiency virus (HIV): The causative virus in AIDS.

Human leucocyte antigen (HLA) testing: A blood test to see whether a person carries a specific gene.

Humoral immune system: One of the two major parts of the immune system. It makes the immunoglobulins that fight infection.

Hyperparathyroidism: A condition caused by low vitamin D levels that predisposes a person to osteoporosis.

Hyperthyroidism: A condition in which an overactive thyroid causes diarrhea, weight loss, palpitations, and intolerance to heat. Also known as Graves' disease.

Hyposplenism: A condition in which an underactive spleen predisposes a person to certain infections.

Hypotonia: Muscle weakness; the "floppiness" seen in a child.

I

Ileum: The last part of the small intestine, found just before the colon.

Immunoglobulin: A bodily protein that fights infection and mediates inflammation.

Immunoglobulin A (IgA): A type of immunoglobulin that is used to test for celiac disease. It is absent in individuals with selective IgA deficiency.

Immunomodulators: Drugs used to treat autoimmune diseases that suppress the immune system.

Immunosuppressant: See Immunomodulators.

Imodium: A drug used to treat diarrhea.

Imuran: A drug that suppresses inflammation and the immune system. It is used to treat autoimmune disease. Also known as azathioprine.

Informed consent: A form signed by the patient or his or her medical proxy that acknowledges the risks and benefits associated with a medical procedure.

Intestinal lymphoma: A cancer of the lymph nodes involving the small intestine. Also known as enteropathy-associated T-cell lymphoma.

Intrauterine growth retardation: Delayed fetal growth.

Intravenous (IV) line: The placement of a needle in the patient's blood vessel, which is then used to infuse fluid into the patient's bloodstream.

Iron: A mineral stored in the body that is used to make hemoglobin, the protein that carries oxygen. Low iron levels can cause anemia.

Iron-deficiency anemia: A type of anemia caused by depleted iron stores.

Irritable bowel syndrome (IBS): A common intestinal disorder characterized by cramps and altered bowel habits (constipation, diarrhea, or both).

J

Jaundice: The symptoms of turning yellow and having dark, tea-colored urine that occur in conjunction with liver disease or hepatitis.

Jejunum: The middle part of the small intestine.

K

Kamut: A gluten-containing grain.

L

Lactase: An enzyme produced in the small intestine that digests the sugar lactose found in cow's milk.

Lactose: A sugar in cow's milk that can cause symptoms for those individuals with lactose intolerance.

Lactose breath test: A test for lactose intolerance.

Lactose intolerance: A common disorder characterized by the loss of the ability to digest lactose. Symptoms include cramps, diarrhea, and gas.

Large intestine: The colon.

Latent celiac disease: An asymptomatic type of celiac disease in which the patient generally has a normal small intestinal biopsy.

Leaky gut: Inflammation of the intestine that promotes leakiness of the gut lining, thereby allowing foreign proteins in.

Liver: An organ in the abdomen that processes nutrients, makes bile, has immune function, and makes proteins.

Lomotil: A prescription medication used to treat diarrhea.

Low-gluten host: A modified communion wafer that contains a small amount of gluten.

Low-residue diet: A diet with a roughage restriction.

Lymphoma: A cancer generally affecting the lymph nodes that can involve any part of the body.

M

Maise: A gluten-free grain.

Malabsorption: The impaired absorption of consumed nutrients.

Malnutrition: A disease of inadequate nutrition, caused by either lack of access to food or impaired food absorption.

Marsh levels: The system used to grade the inflammation seen under the microscope in biopsies with celiac disease.

Matzo flour/meal: A gluten-containing flour.

Melanocyte: A cell generally found in the skin that produces pigment.

Mesquite: A gluten-free flour.

Metamucil: A fiber supplement used to regulate bowel movements.

Microscopic colitis: A type of inflammation of the colon that causes diarrhea and can be identified via biopsy.

Milk of magnesia: A laxative medication used to treat constipation.

Millet: A gluten-free grain.

Miralax: A type of laxative commonly used to prepare the bowel for a colonoscopy.

Montina: A gluten-free starch.

Mortality: Death rate.

Mucosa: The lining of the intestine.

Myasthenia gravis: An autoimmune disease of muscle causing weakness.

Myopathy: An inflammatory condition affecting the muscles.

N

Neuropathy: An inflammatory condition of nerves that is accompanied by numbness and tingling of the arms and legs.

Nonclassical celiac disease: Celiac disease with atypical or no manifestations.

Non-Hodgkin's lymphoma (NHL): A type of lymphoma.

Non-tropical sprue: Another name for celiac disease.

O

Oats: A type of grain that when "pure" may be tolerated on a gluten-free diet.

Obesity: The condition of being overweight by about 30 pounds. Obesity increases a person's risk of cancer, stroke, diabetes, and heart disease.

Omega-3 fatty acid: A type of oil generally found in fish that decreases inflammation.

Orzo: A gluten-containing pasta.

Osmotically active: The condition in which a substance draws water into the gut.

Osteopenia: Mild thinning of the bones. It is treated with calcium and vitamin D supplements.

Osteoporosis: Severe thinning of the bone with increased risk of fractures.

P

Pancreatic islet cells: The cells that make insulin.

Panko: A gluten-containing food additive.

Parathyroid gland: A gland located in the neck that produces parathyroid hormone.

Parathyroid hormone: A blood hormone whose level is elevated in osteoporosis and vitamin D deficiency.

PEP: A type of enzyme being studied as a treatment for celiac disease.

Perforation: A hole in the wall of the intestine that requires surgery to repair.

Peripheral neuropathy: Numbness or tingling in the arms and legs.

Pernicious anemia: A vitamin B_{12} deficiency that results in anemia.

Pimecrolimus (Elidel): A medication used to treat inflammatory conditions of the skin.

Pneumococcal vaccine: A vaccine against a type of pneumonia.

Potato starch/flour: A gluten-free starch.

Potential celiac disease: See Latent celiac disease.

Prealbumin: A protein produced by the liver that is a marker of nutritional status.

Prednisone: A steroid medication used to suppress inflammation.

Primary biliary cirrhosis: A chronic inflammatory condition of the liver that tends to occur in women and may be associated with celiac disease.

Primary sclerosing cholangitis: A chronic inflammatory condition of the liver characterized by scarring of the bile ducts.

Probiotics: Supplements that increase the number of beneficial bacteria in the intestine.

Protein: A nitrogen-containing substance that is made up of amino acids.

Psoriasis: An inflammatory condition of the skin characterized by thick, scaly plaques.

Pyx: The vessel used to store the wafer host in communion.

Q

Quinoa: A gluten-free starch.

R

Refractory (sprue) celiac disease: Celiac disease that does not respond to a gluten-free diet.

Rheumatoid arthritis: An autoimmune arthritis that causes joint inflammation and destruction.

Rheumatologist: A doctor who specializes in the treatment of muscle, bone, and joint diseases.

Rice: A gluten-free grain.

Rickets: A vitamin D deficiency found in children with malformed bones.

Rye: A gluten-containing grain.

S

Sago: A gluten-free grain.

Scalloping of the mucosa: An abnormality seen on endoscopic examination of the duodenum; it requires biopsy to confirm celiac disease.

Scleroderma: An autoimmune inflammatory condition that can affect any part of the body and is characterized by thickening and scarring of the affected part.

Scurvy: A vitamin C deficiency that is manifested as bruising and hair and tooth loss.

Secretin: A synthetic hormone used in gastrointestinal testing that has variable benefits for autism.

Sedimentation rate (ESR): A blood test for inflammation.

Seitan: A toxic gluten-containing wheat derivative.

Selective immunoglobulin A (IgA) deficiency: The most common immunodeficiency, caused by inability to produce IgA.

Semolina: A gluten-containing wheat.

Sensitivity: The ability of a test to detect a true positive result.

Sicca syndrome: An autoimmune syndrome characterized by dry eyes and mouth and caused by destruction of glands.

Silent celiac disease: Asymptomatic celiac disease.

Sjogren's syndrome: An autoimmune disease of the tear glands and salivary glands that results in dry eyes and mouth.

Small bowel follow-through: A barium x-ray of the small intestine.

Small intestinal bacterial overgrowth (SIBO): Overgrowth of the number and type of bacteria in the small intestine, causing diarrhea, weight loss, and vitamin deficiencies.

Small intestine: The site of digestion and absorption of nutrients.

Small intestine biopsy: A biopsy taken at the time of endoscopy for the purpose of making the diagnosis of celiac disease.

Smooth muscle: The muscle in the lining of the intestine that moves materials forward in the gut.

Sorghum: A gluten-free starch.

Soy: A gluten-free starch. It is not equivalent to soy sauce.

Specificity: The ability of a test to pick up a true positive result.

Spelt: A gluten-containing wheat.

Spleen: An organ in the left upper part of the abdomen that protects the body against infection.

Sprue: Another name for celiac disease.

Steroids: Medications used to treat inflammation.

Stricture: A narrowing of the intestine.

Surreptitious gluten ingestion: Ingestion of gluten from an unknown source.

T

Tacrolimus (Protopic): An anti-inflammatory medication used to treat some skin conditions.

Tapioca: A gluten-free starch.

Teff: A gluten-free flour.

Tetany: A spasm of the muscles caused by very low blood calcium levels.

Thiamine: An essential vitamin that can be deficient in celiac disease.

Thyroid: A gland in the neck that is the body's thermostat and controls metabolism.

Tight junctions: The protein structures that hold together the cells that line the small intestine.

Tissue transglutaminase antibody (tTG): A blood test commonly used to screen for celiac disease.

Total parenteral nutrition (TPN): Intravenous feeding used when the gut has failed.

Transferrin: A blood protein that is a marker of nutritional status.

Trisomy 21: See Down syndrome.

Triticale: A gluten-containing wheat.

Tropical sprue: An infectious disease of the small intestine that mimics celiac disease and is treated with antibiotics.

T-score: The scoring scale for bone density scans. It is used to diagnose osteoporosis.

Tuberculosis: A chronic infectious disease that requires prolonged antibiotics for treatment.

Turner syndrome: A syndrome present a birth that affects females and is highly associated with celiac disease.

Type 1 diabetes: An autoimmune disease of the pancreas that affects children. It is often associated with celiac disease.

U

Ulcerative jejunitis: A refractory type of celiac disease that can evolve into lymphoma.

Undiagnosed celiac disease: The presence of symptoms without a diagnosis that is eventually recognized as celiac disease.

Upper GI series: An x-ray examination of the small intestine.

V

Villi: The finger-like projections that line the small intestine and are the sites of digestion and absorption of food.

Vitamin A: A fat-soluble vitamin required for vision and skin health.

Vitamin B$_{12}$: A vitamin required for blood production and nerve and brain function. A deficiency of B$_{12}$ can require monthly vitamin shots.

Vitamin C: A vitamin found in citrus fruits that is required for wound healing and skin integrity.

Vitamin D: A fat-soluble vitamin found in dairy products that maintains bone health.

Vitamin K: A fat-soluble vitamin made by intestinal bacteria that helps to clot blood.

Vitiligo: An autoimmune skin condition characterized by patchy loss of pigmentation with white spots.

VSL #3: A commercially available probiotic supplement of beneficial bacteria.

W

Warfarin (Coumadin): A drug used to thin the blood, thereby preventing blood clots.

Wheat bran/germ/starch: Gluten-containing wheat products.

Whipple's disease: An infectious disease of the small intestine characterized by gastrointestinal and neurologic symptoms.

Williams syndrome: A rare genetic disorder of mental retardation that is highly associated with celiac disease.

Z

Zinc: An essential mineral that maintains the body's wound-healing ability.

Zonulin: A protein that helps regulate the movement of nutrients into the cells lining the villi.

INDEX

Index

page numbers followed by *f* denote figures; those followed by *t* denote tables

Absorption, 2, 195
Addison's disease, 166*f*
Additives to food that may contain gluten, 122*t*, 128*t*
Adenocarcinoma, 175, 195
Albumin, 195
Alcohol, gluten-free, 121–122, 121*t*
Algorithm for celiac blood testing, 80*f*
Allergies to food
    relation to CD and, 9–11
    and sensitivity to gluten, compared, 46–47
Alopecia areata, 158–159, 166*f*, 195
Amaranth, 195
Ambulatory endoscopy center, 86, 195
Amenorrhea, 36, 195
American College of Gastroenterology patient information on CD, 188, 188*t*
Amino acids, 2, 195
Anaphylaxis, 11, 195
Anemia, 8, 16–17, 22*t*, 33–36
    causes of
        abnormal production of red blood cells, 34–36
        loss of red blood cells (bleeding), 34
        shortened red blood cell lifespan, 36
    complete blood count (CBC), 33–34
    definition of, 195
    general symptoms of, 33
Anesthesia, during endoscopy, 88–89
Animal models, development of, 190–191
Antibody-negative patients with CD, diagnosis for, 81–82
Antiendomysial antibody (EMA) test, 61, 70, 74–77, 77*t*
    annual testing, 144–145
    definition of, 195
Antigliadin antibody (AGA) test, 70, 74, 75, 77, 77*t*
    definition of, 195
    usefulness of, 81–82
Antispasmodic drugs, 29, 30*t*, 195
Aphthous stomatitis (mouth sores or ulcers), 18, 65, 158*t*, 166*f*, 195
Arrowroot, 195
Arthritis and bone pain, 19
AT-1001, 112, 192, 195
Ataxia, 18–19, 37–38, 195
Atrophic gastritis, 166*f*
Atropine, 30*t*
Atypical celiac disease, 19–20, 195
Autism and CD, 58–59
    definition of autism, 196
    gluten-free and casein-free diet, 59
    leaky gut hypothesis, 59
    secretin therapy for autism, 58
Autoimmune disease

associated with CD, 21–22, 22*t*,
166*f*
factors in development of, 165
rate of, 165
in children, 57
definition of, 2, 3, 196
manifestations of, 164–165
Autoimmune hepatitis (AIH), 41, 196
Autoimmune liver diseases, 41,
42, 196. *See also* Liver disease
associated with CD
Autoimmune thyroid disease, 45, 60*t*
Azathioprine, 173, 196

B vitamin deficiency, in children with
CD, 66*t*
Bacteria, beneficial, 152–153, 196
Bacterial overgrowth, 22*t*, 23, 116, 196
described, 145–146
empiric treatment for, 147
symptoms, 141
testing for, 146–147
Barium studies, 98–100, 99*f*, 196
Barley, 2, 3, 196
Barley extract (barley malt), 196
Bay Area Celiacs, 183*t*
Belfast, Ireland, adults, rate of CD
among, 6*t*
Benedictine Sisters of Clyde, 130
Beneficial bacteria, 152–153, 196
Bentyl (dicyclomine), 30*t*
Bile, 45, 196
Bile salt diarrhea, 45, 50, 196
Biopsy
definition of, 196
orienting the biopsy technique,
85–86
skin, diagnosis of DH, 159
small intestine, diagnosis of CD, 5,
6, 54, 61–62, 204

changes seen in other diseases,
94–95
changes seen in the biopsy of CD,
93–95
Marsh levels, 94, 94*f*
confirming the diagnosis, 95
functions of the small intestine
and villi, 91–93, 92*f*
purpose of, 89–90
safety of, 90
second opinions, 95
Bisphosphonates, 40, 148, 196
Bleeding risk, during endoscopy, 88
Blood testing for CD
abnormalities associated with CD,
23–24, 24*t*
algorithm for celiac blood testing,
80*f*
for children, 61–62
problems associated with blood
testing
false-negative results because of
IgA deficiency, 79–81
inappropriate physician
interpretation of results, 78
inconsistency of results, 79
patients who have no positive
tests, 81
recommended tests
antiendomysial antibody (EMA)
test, 74–77, 77*t*
antigliadin antibody (AGA) test,
77, 77*t*
avoiding potential for false-
positive results, 78
concepts of sensitivity and
specificity, 75–76, 75*t*
single needle stick or blood draw,
76
tissue transglutaminase (tTG)
test, 77, 77*t*

Body mass index (BMI), 24–25, 136, 196
Bone density scan, 39, 40, 102, 103, 147–148, 196
Bone disease. See Osteopenia; Osteoporosis
Bone growth, in children with CD, 64
Bone mineral density (BMD), 64, 196
Boniva, 40
Books on celiac disease, 193
Bowel obstruction, 98, 196
Breath test, 31–32, 146, 147, 201
Buckwheat, 196
Budesonide, 173, 196
Bulgur, 196

C-reative protein (CPR), 197
Calcium
  blood levels, 40, 102–103, 104t
  deficiency in children with CD, 64–65, 66t
  role of, 149t
  supplementation, 40, 150t
Caltrate, 40
Canadian Celiac Association, 183t
Canadians, rate of CD among, 6t
Cancer, 42–43, 67, 137, 174–176
Capsule endoscopy ("PillCam"), 95–98, 197
  the capsule endoscope, 96f
  limitations, 97–98
  procedure, 97
  risk of bowel obstruction, 98
Carotene (Vitamin A)
  definition of, 197
  test, 104
Case, Shelley, 110
Casein-free diet
  for autistic children, 59
  definition of, 197

CAT scans, diagnosis of neurological abnormalities, 37
Catholic Celiac Society, 131
Celiac disease (CD), overview
  definition of, 2–4, 197
  diagnosis of, 5 (See also Evaluation and diagnosis)
  does it affect both genders?, 8
  the future of CD
    development of an animal model, 190–191
    increased education for healthcare professionals, 191
    potential therapies, 191–192
    research into potential medications for CD, 191
    targets for investigation, 190
  genes that predispose a person to having CD, 7
  history of, 4–5
  incidence of among ethnic groups, 5–6, 6t
  is it related to other food allergies, 9–11
  other names for CD, 2–4, 8–9
  rates of CD among relatives, 6–8, 7t
  types of
    atypical CD, 19–20
    classic, 19
    collagenous sprue, 21
    latent CD, 20
    refractory (sprue) celiac disease, 21
    silent CD, 20
    surreptitious gluten ingestion, 20
    undiagnosed CD, 20
Celiac Disease Foundation, 183t, 187t
Celiac Disease On-line Support, 183t

Celiac Disease Support Group at
Children's Hospital Boston, 187*t*
Celiac-friendly stores, 119, 120*t*
Celiac panel of tests, 75
Celiac patient support groups,
182–184, 183*t*
Celiac sprue. *See* Celiac disease (CD)
Celiac Sprue Association (CSA)
Gluten-Free Product Listing, 110,
115
motto, 192
websites, 183*t*, 185*t*
Celiac Support Groups in the U.S.,
183*t*, 187*t*
Celiac website for children, 187*t*
Celiac.com, 187*t*
Cellular immune system, 74, 197
Chickpea, 197
Children and celiac disease
the autism link, 58–59
complications of CD
affects of symptoms and chronic
discomfort, 64
effects of other vitamin and
mineral deficiencies, 65, 66*t*
effects of vitamin D and calcium
malabsorption, 64–65
neurologic, 66
other autoimmune diseases, 66–67
risk of cancer, 67
risk of obesity, 67
stunting of bone growth, 64
type 1 diabetes and its
complications, 65–66
diagnostic testing for CD in
children, 61–62
diseases associated with CD in
children
associated diseases

dermatitis herpetiformis (DH),
57
other autoimmune diseases, 57
Sjogren's syndrome, 57
Type 1 (juvenile) diabetes, 57
genetic diseases
Down syndrome, 55–56
selective IgA deficiency, 56–57
Turner syndrome, 56
Williams syndrome, 56
recommended testing for tTG,
57–58
do children get CD?, 52–53
manifestations of CD in, 15
classical CD, 53, 55*t*
latent or potential CD, 54, 54*f*
nonclassical CD, 53, 55*t*
silent CD, 53, 54*f*
symptomatic CD, 54, 54*f*
rate of CD in children, 52–53
ratio of asymptomatic to
symptomatic children, 53, 54
screening children for CD
first-degree relatives, 60
guidelines, 59
high-risk children, 60, 60*t*
support or information for, 186–
187, 187*t*
treatment: the gluten-free diet
follow-up with a physician, 64
issues, 63
recovery from latent CD in
children on the diet, 137–138
strategies for adherance to, 63
vitamin and mineral supplements,
63–64
Chronic hepatitis, 166*f*
Cincinnati Celiac Support Group,
183*t*
Cincinnati ROCK, 187*t*

Cirrhosis, 41, 166f, 197
Citracal, 40
Citrucil, 28, 29, 197
Classic celiac disease
    in children, 53, 55t
    definition of, 19, 197
Clidinium (Librax), 30t
Clopidogrel (Plavix), 197
"Coeliac Affection," 52
Colitis, microscopic, 22t, 23
Collagen, 172, 197
Collagenous sprue, 21, 172, 197
Colon, 44, 197
Colonoscopy, 45–46, 101
Communion wafer (host) and other
    gluten-containing religious
    products, 129–131
Complete blood count (CBC), 33–34,
    104t, 197
Complications. See also Diseases
    associated with CD
CD and cancer (including lymphoma),
    relationship between, 174–176
    in children, 64–67
    collagenous sprue, 172
    gluten-free diet to prevent
        complications of CD, 136,
        176–177
    obesity, 177–179
    refractory sprue, 172–173
    risk of mortality, 176
    small intestinal lymphoma, 174
    ulcerative jejunitis, 173–174
Corn, 197
Couscous, 197
Crohn's disease, 8, 48, 197
CT scans, 102

Dapsone (sulfapyridine), 160, 197
Death rate, patients with CD, 42

Dental enamel, 18, 197
Depression, in patients with CD, 38
Dermal papillae, 159, 198
Dermatitis herpetiformis (DH), 18,
        22t 60t, 73
    age of onset, 156
    association with other autoimmune
        diseases, 156
    in children, 57
    definition of, 198
    described, 156
    diagnosis of, 157, 159
    genetic transmission of: HLA-
        DQ2and HLA-DQ8 genes, 156,
        157
    other skin diseases associated with
        CD, 158–159, 158t
    relationship between DH and CD,
        157
    symptoms of, 157
    treatment, 160
DEXA scan. See also Bone density
        scan
    definition of, 198
Diabetes, Type 1 (juvenile). See Type 1
        (juvenile) diabetes
Diagnosis of CD. See Evaluation and
        diagnosis
Diarrhea
    in children, 15
    diarrheal diseases occurring with
        CD, 14, 43–46
    causes of
        autoimmune thyroid disease, 45
        bile salt diarrhea, 45
        irritable bowel syndrome, 44
        lactose intolerance, 44
        microscopic colitis, 45–46
        small intestine bacterial
            overgrowth (SIBO), 44–45

evaluation by a colonoscopy, 45–46
frequent, low-residue diet for, 10
Dicke, Willem, 4–5, 52
Dicyclomine (Bentyl), 30*t*
Dietitians, 109–110
role of in the gluten-free diet, 184–185
education about the diet, 112
identifying potential problem areas in the diet, 113
managing weight issues, 113
providing a balanced diet, 113–114
strategies to avoid gluten in your diet, 112
Digestion, 2, 198
Dinkle, 198
Diseases associated with CD
anemia, 33–36
autoimmune disease, 164–165, 166*f*
in children
dermatitis herpetiformis (DH), 57
genetic diseases
Down syndrome, 55–56
selective IgA deficiency, 56–57
Turner syndrome, 56
Williams syndrome, 56
other autoimmune diseases, 57
Sjogren's syndrome, 57
Type 1 (juvenile) diabetes, 57
Endocrine diseases, 166*f*
gastrointestinal disease, 166*f*
liver disease, 166*f*, 168–170, 169*t*
neurological disease, 18–19, 37–38, 66, 166*f*
rheumatologic disease, 166*f*
selective IgA deficiency, 162–163
skin diseases, 158–159, 158*t*, 166*f*
alopecia areata, 158–159
dermatitis herpetiformis (DH), 156–160
eczema, 158
psoriasis, 158
vitiligo, 158
thyroid disease, 166–168
type 1 diabetes, 163–164
Diseases that mimic CD
bile salt diarrhea, 50
Crohn's disease, 48
giardia, 49
gluten sensitivity, 47
HIV, 49
hyperthyroidism, 49
IBS, 47
microscopic colitis, 48
tropical sprue, 48
tuberculosis, 49
Whipple's disease, 48
Donnatal (phenobarbital), 30*t*
Down syndrome, 22, 22*t*, 55–56, 60*t*, 198
Dry beri beri, 38, 198
Dry mouth, 22*t*
Duodenum, 34, 35*f*, 198
Durum, 198

EATL. *See* Enteropathy-associated T-cell lymphoma (EATL)
Eczema, 18, 22*t*, 158, 166*f*, 198
Education for healthcare professionals about CD, 191
Einkorn, 198
Elidel (pimecrolimus), 160
Emmer, 198
Encephalopathy, 37–38, 198
Endocrine diseases associated with CD, 166*f*
Endocrinologist, 40, 198
Endoscope, 86

Endoscopy, 5, 198
  ambulatory endoscopy center, 86
  in children, 62
  the endoscope, 86
  pain associated with, 88–89
  preparation for the test, 86–87
  procedure, 87–88
  recovery, 88
  samples from the villi, 86
Enteropathy-associated T-cell
    lymphoma (EATL), 43
  definition of, 198
  evaluation, 175
  risk for, 176
  symptoms, 175
  treatment for, 175–176
Environmental sources of gluten,
    126–127
Enzyme supplements, 32, 110, 111
Enzymes, 198
EP-B2 enzyme, 111, 198
Evaluation and diagnosis, 5
  antigliadin test, usefulness of, 81–82
  barium studies, 98–100, 99f
  biopsy of the small intestine
    changes seen in other diseases,
      94–95
    changes seen in the biopsy of CD,
      93–95
      Marsh levels, 94, 94f
    confirming the diagnosis, 95
    functions of the small intestine
      and villi, 91–93, 92f
    purpose of, 89–90
    safety of, 90
    second opinions, 95
  capsule endoscopy (PillCam"),
      95–98
    the capsule endoscope, 96f
    limitations, 97–98

procedure, 97
    risk of bowel obstruction, 98
  diagnosis for antibody-negative
    patients with CD, 81–82
  diagnosis for CD patients with
    negative blood tests, 81
  endoscopy test
    ambulatory endoscopy center, 86
    pain associated with, 88–89
    preparation for the test, 86–87
    procedure, 87–88
    recovery, 88
    samples from the villi, 86
  how CD is diagnosed
    biopsies of small intestine mucosa,
      70–71
    blood testing, 70, 75
    false-negative results, 71
    methods not used for diagnosis,
      71
  human leucocyte antigen (HLA)
    testing
    confirming or ruling out a
      diagnosis of CD with, 83, 84
    genes associated with, 83–84
  other tests
    blood tests, non-CD-specific, 102
    colonoscopy with biopsy, 101
    CT or MRI scans, 102
    stool studies, 100–101
  problems associated with blood
    testing
    algorithm for celiac blood testing,
      80f
    false-negative results because of
      IgA deficiency, 79–81
    inappropriate physician
      interpretation of results, 78
    inconsistency of results, 79

patients who have no positive tests, 81

recommended blood testing
   antiendomysial antibody (EMA) test, 74–77, 77*t*
   antigliadin antibody (AGA) test, 77, 77*t*
   avoiding potential for false-positive results, 78
   concepts of sensitivity and specificity, 75–76, 75*t*
   single needle stick or blood draw, 76
   tissue transglutaminase (tTG) test, 77, 77*t*

seeing a gastroenterologist, 71–72

small intestinal biopsy ("gold standard" test for CD)
   "orienting the biopsy" technique, 85–86
   patients must be on a gluten-free diet, 85
   processing the tissue samples, 85

symptoms which warrant testing for CD, 72–74
   anemia or osteoporosis, 73
   asymptomatic family members of person with CD, 73
   atypical symptoms, 73
   dermatitis herpetiformis (DH), 73
   gastrointestinal symptoms and weight loss, 72–73
   other autoimmune diseases, 73

tests performed after new diagnosis of CD, 102–104, 104*t*
   bone density scan, 103
   carotene level, 104
   vitamin and mineral levels, 102–103, 104

understanding the immune system, 74–75

False-negative blood test results, 71, 79–81, 163

False-positive blood test results, 78

Farina, 198

Faro, 198

Fat-soluble vitamins, 38, 39, 198. *See also* specific vitamins, A, D, and K

Fatty liver disease, 22*t*, 41, 42, 198

Fava, 198

Female-to-male ratio for having CD, 8

Fermentum, 130, 198

Ferritin, 199

Finnish students, rate of CD among, 6*t*

First-degree relative, 6, 7, 7*t*, 60*tt*, 199

Fish oil (omega-3 fatty acid) supplementation, 152, 153–154, 199

Flax, 199

Flu shot, 151, 199

Folic acid (folate) deficiency, 36, 104*t*, 145, 199

Food additives that may contain gluten, 122*t*, 128*t*

Foods, possibly contaminated with gluten, 128*t*

Fosamax, 40

Gastroenterologist, 43, 71–72, 199

Gastrointestinal disease associated with CD, 166*f*

Gastrointestinal symptoms associated with CD, 14–15, 15*t*

Gee, Samuel, 52

Gender, female-to-male ratio for having CD, 8

Genes

associated with CD, 7, 54, 83–84, 156, 157
definition of, 83, 199
Genetic diseases associated with CD in children
Down syndrome, 55–56
selective IgA deficiency, 56–57
Turner syndrome, 56
Williams syndrome, 56
Genetic disorder, definition of, 3, 4, 199
Giardia, 49, 199
Gluten. *See also under* Gluten-free diet
-containing grains, 107–108, 108*t*
-containing ingredients, checking labels for, 106
definition of, 2, 3, 106, 199
first found to be the cause of CD, 52
in medications, 106–107
Gluten-free diet
alcohol consumption and, 121–122, 121*t*
for autistic children, 59
for autoimmune thyroid disease, 167
benefits of
complete recovery from latent CD in children, 137–138
correction of nutritional deficiencies, 136
improvement of symptoms, 136
prevention of celiac-associated complications, 136
reduction in risk of lymphoma, 137
reduction in risk of refractory sprue and death, 137
benefits to children with CD, 66, 67

causes of symptoms after starting the diet
bacterial overgrowth, 116
continued consumption of gluten, 115
microscopic colitis requiring medication, 116–117
surreptitious consumption of gluten, 115–116
causes of symptoms after years on the diet, 117
communion wafer (host) and other gluten-containing religious products, 129–131
definition of, 199
for DH, 160
dietary trials of, 131–132
food additives that may contain gluten, 122*t*
gluten-free grains and starches, 114–115, 114*t*
gluten-free multivitamins, 114
irritable bowel syndrome (IBS) and, 132–133
is it for life?
asymptomatic patients with an immune response, 139
patients who are willing to suffer the consequences, 139–140
patients who do not have the capacity to understand the diet, 140
is there a medication or pill to cure CD?, 110–112
action of zonulin in the intestines, 111–112
combination enzyme therapy and enzyme supplements, 110
medication-related studies, 110–111

oats in the diet, 118–119
prior to blood testing or intestinal
  biopsies, 62, 85
recurring symptoms with a gluten
  exposure after starting the diet,
  138–139
resources for information on, 183t,
  184–186
restaurants that are celiac-friendly,
  122–123, 124–125t, 126
results of unknown gluten
  ingestion, 139
role of the dietitian
  education about the diet, 112
  identifying potential problem
  areas in the diet, 113
  managing weight issues, 113
  providing a balanced diet,
  113–114
  strategies to avoid gluten in your
  diet, 112
sources of gluten contamination
  dietary gluten, 127–129
    food additives, 128t
    possibly contaminated foods,
    128t
  environmental and nondietary
  sources, 126–127
vendors of gluten-free foods, 119,
  120t
what is it?
  "gluten-free" defined for the U.S.,
  109
  meeting with a dietitian for
  information, 109–110
  need for with potential or latent
  CD, 110
  prescribed by doctors for allergy
  to gluten proteins, 108
  resources for information, 110

a true gluten-free diet, 108–109
Gluten-Free Diet, 110, 185t
"Gluten-free diet guide for families,"
  185t
Gluten Free in WNY, 183t
Gluten-Free Mall, 185t
Gluten-Free Oats, 118
Gluten-Free Product Listing (CSA),
  110, 115
Gluten Intolerance Group, 109, 183t
Gluten-sensitive enteropathy. See
  Celiac disease (CD)
Gluten sensitivity, 9, 199
  and allergy, compared, 46–47
Glycolax, 29, 199
Gold standard test for CD. See under
  Biopsy
Graham flour, 199
Grains
  gluten-containing, 107–108, 108t
  gluten-free grains and starches,
  114–115, 114t
Graves' disease (hyperthyroidism), 22t,
  39, 49, 199
  definition of, 200
  physical signs of, 167
  treatment, 167
Great Northern Growers, Montana,
  118

Hashimoto's thyroiditis (disease), 22t,
  199
  symptoms and treatment of, 167
Healthy Villi (Boston area), 183t
Hematocrit (HCT) test, 16, 33, 199
Hemoglobin (Hb) test, 16, 33, 199
Hepatitis, 40, 41, 166f, 199
  testing and vaccination for hepatitis
  A and B, 152

High-risk populations, rates of CD in, 60, 60*t*
HLA-DQ2/HLA-DQ8 genes, 7, 54, 83–84, 156, 157, 199
Host, 129–131, 200
Human immunodeficiency virus (HIV), 49, 200
Human leucocyte antigen (HLA) testing, 200
    confirming or ruling out a diagnosis of CD with, 83, 84
    genes associated with, 83–84
Humoral immune system, 74–75, 200
Hyoscyamine (Levsin, Nulex, Levbid, Pamine), 30*t*
Hyperparathyroidism, 200
Hyperthyroidism. *See* Graves' disease (hyperthyroidism)
Hyposplenism, 151, 200
Hypothyroidism. *See* Hashimoto's thyroiditis (disease)
Hypotonia, 66, 200

Ileum, 35, 35*f*, 200
Immune response, inflammation, 138, 153–154
Immune system, 74–75
Immunoglobulin A (IgA), 200. *See also* Selective immunoglobulin A (IgA) deficiency
Immunoglobulins, 79, 200
Immunomodulators (immunosuppressants), 173, 200
Imodium, 29, 116, 200
Imuran, 173, 200
Incidence of CD
    among ethnic groups, 5–6, 6*t*
    among relatives, 6–8, 7*t*
Incontinence of stools, 14
Infection risk, after endoscopy, 89

Inflammation
    gluten ingestion and, 138
    omega-3 fatty acid supplementation and, 153–154
Informed consent, 89, 200
Intestinal lymphoma, 200. See also under Lymphoma
Intestine
    large, 44
    small
        biopsy of (*See under* Biopsy)
        definition of, 2
        work of, 14
Intrauterine growth retardation, 37, 200
Intravenous (IV) line, 87, 200
Iron, 8, 21
    definition of, 200
    role of, 149*t*
    supplementation, 150*t*
    testing for iron status, 104*t*
Iron-deficiency anemia, 34, 73, 136, 200
Irritable bowel syndrome (IBS), 9, 44, 47, 200
    causes of, 28
    and checking for CD, 27–28, 30
    described, 27
    does a gluten-free diet help?, 132–133
    initial treatment, 28–29, 142
    medications for, 29, 30*t*
    post-infectious IBS, 28
    symptoms, 142
Italian school children, rate of CD among, 6*t*

Jaundice, 40, 41, 200
Jejunum, 34, 35*f*, 201

Juvenile (Type 1) diabetes. *See* Type 1 (juvenile) diabetes

Kamut, 201

Lactaid/Lactaid Ultra, 32
Lactase, 10, 142, 201
Lactose, 10, 142, 201
Lactose breath test, 31–32, 146, 147, 201
Lactose intolerance, 44
   association with CD, 31
   in certain ethnic groups, 31
   in children, 30–31
   definition of, 10, 201
   description of, 30, 141
   diagnosis of by a breath test, 31–32, 146, 147, 201
   diagnosis of by its symptoms, 31
   dietary restrictions, 31
   should all people with it be checked for CD?, 32–33
   treatment, 32
Large intestine, 44, 201
Latent (potential) CD, 20, 201
   in children, 54, 54*f*, 137–138
   need to follow a gluten-free diet or not, 110
Leaky gut, 59, 112, 201
Librium (Librax), 30*t*
Liver, 40, 201
Liver disease associated with CD, 166*f*
   "cryptogenic" chronic liver disease, 169
   percent of transplant patients with CD, 168
   risk of developing CD, patients with preexisting liver disease, 168, 169*t*
   risk of developing liver disease, patients with preexisting CD, 168, 169*t*
   testing and vaccination for hepatitis A and B, 152
   testing for, 169–170
Liver function tests (LFTs), 104*t*
Lomotil, 29, 201
Low-gluten host, guidelines, 130–131, 201
Low-residue diet, 10, 11, 201
Lupus, 22*t*, 166*f*
Lymphoma, 42–43
   definition of, 201
   enteropathy-associated T-cell lymphoma (EATL)
   evaluation, 175
   symptoms, 175
   treatment for, 175–176
   overall risk of, 137
   small intestinal, 174, 175
   symptoms, 141

Magnesium
   role of, 149*t*
   supplementation, 150*t*
Magnetic resonance imaging (MRI), 38, 102
Maise, 201
Malabsorption, 2, 3, 15, 201
Malnutrition, 19, 201
Management of CD. *See also* Gluten-free diet
   annual EMA and tTG blood testing, 144–145
   bacterial overgrowth, 145–147
   bone density scan (DXA/DEXA), 147–148
   fish oil (omega-3) or probiotic supplementation, 151–153

the gluten-free diet: benefits of
complete recovery from latent
CD in children, 137–138
correction of nutritional
deficiencies, 136
improvement of symptoms, 136
prevention of celiac-associated
complications, 136
reduction in risk of lymphoma,
137
reduction in risk of refractory
sprue and death, 137
the gluten-free diet: is it for life?
asymptomatic patients with an
immune response, 139
patients who are willing to suffer
the consequences, 139–140
patients who do not have the
capacity to understand the diet,
140
recurring symptoms with a gluten
exposure after starting the diet,
138–139
results of unknown gluten
ingestion, 139
the gluten-free diet: when it isn't
working, 140–141
other foods that need to be avoided,
141–142
role of the physician in diagnosis
annual testing for patients with
CD, 144*t*
evaluating weight loss or gain, 143
evaluation and instruction by a
dietitian, 143–144
initial testing, 143
observation of symptoms and
response to the diet, 142–143
vaccinations, 151–152

vitamin and mineral
supplementation, 149–150, 149*t*,
150*t*
Marsh levels, 94, 94*f*, 201
Marye's story
antiendomysial blood test, 24
avoiding grains, 108
bone density test, 40
celiac disease, 4, 7–8
celiac-friendly stores, 120
comments on support groups and
information for CD patients, 184,
186, 187
the endoscopy test, 90
food choices today, 53
gastrointestinal symptoms, 16
gluten-free alcohol, 122
gluten-free diet, 138
gluten-free restaurant menus, 126
liver function tests, 42
oats in her diet, 119
read labels for gluten-containing
ingredients, 107
receiving communion, 131
symptoms even with the gluten-
free diet, 117
vitamin supplementation, 150
Matzo/flour/meal, 201
Mayo clinic patient information, 188*t*
Medications
anti-inflammatory, 153–154
bisphosphonates, 40, 148, 196
gluten-containing, 106
gluten-free, 107
for IBS, 29, 30*t*
medication-related studies, 110–
111
for microscopic colitis, 116–117
research into potential medications
for CD, 191

treatment of DH, 160
treatment of refractory sprue, 173
MedicineNet.com, 188t
Melanocytes, 158, 201
Mesquite, 201
Metamucil, 28, 201
Microscopic colitis, 45–46, 48
  definition of, 201
  medication for, 116–117
  symptoms, 141
Milk and dairy products, lactose
  intolerance and, 30–32
Milk of magnesia, 29, 201
Millet, 201
Mineral levels in blood, testing for,
  102–103, 104t
Miralax, 29, 201
Montina, 201
Mortality, patients with CD, 42, 176
  mortality defined, 201
MRI (magnetic resonance imaging)
  scans, 38, 102
Mucosa
  definition of, 201
  scalloping of, 90
Multiple sclerosis, 166f
Multivitamins. See also specific
  nutrients
  gluten-free, 114
  and mineral supplementation, 150t
Muscle abnormalities, 19
Myasthenia gravis, 166f, 201
Myopathy, 37–38, 202

NASPGHAN (North American
  Society of Pediatric
  Gastroenterology, Hepatology,
  and Nutrition), 110, 187t
National Digestive Disease Clearing
  House, 188t

National Foundation for Celiac
  Awareness, 183t
National Foundation for Celiac
  Awareness kids corner, 187t
National Institute of Health links on
  CD, 188t
Neurological disease associated with
  CD, 18–19, 37–38, 66, 166f
Neuropathy, 65, 202
Non-Hodgkin's lymphoma (NHL),
  42, 43, 202
Non-tropical sprue. See Celiac disease
  (CD)
Nonclassical CD
  in children, 53, 55t
  definition of, 202
Nondietary sources of gluten, 126–127
North American Society of Pediatric
  Gastroenterology, Hepatology,
  and Nutrition (NASPGHAN),
  110, 187t
Nutritional deficiencies. See also
  specific nutrients
  correcting with a gluten-free diet,
  67

Oats in a gluten-free diet, 118–119,
  202
Obesity and weight gain
  associated with a gluten-free diet,
  177–179
  body mass index (BMI), 24–25
  as complication of CD in children,
  67
  factors contributing to, 25–26
  obesity defined, 202
  and overweight in the United
  States, 24, 25, 26f, 177

Omega-3 fatty acid (fish oil)
   supplementation, 153–154, 199,
   202
Omega-6 fatty acids, 154
Oral manifestations of CD, 18
Orienting the biopsy technique, 85–86
Orzo, 202
Osmotically active, 46–47, 202
Osteopenia, 39, 103, 202
Osteoporosis, 8, 17–18, 22t, 38–40,
   103
   definition of, 202
   evaluation for bone health, 39–40,
      147–148
   low blood calcium levels and, 39
   poor absorption of vitamin D and,
      39, 136
   risk factors, 38–39, 148
   treatments, 39–40, 148

Pain associated with endoscopy, 88–89
Pancreatic islet cells, 164, 202
Pancreatitis, 166f
Panko, 202
Parathyroid gland, 65, 202
Parathyroid hormone, 202
PEP enzyme, 111, 202
Perforation, 175, 202
   risk of, during endoscopy, 88
Peripheral neuropathy, 37–38, 202
Pernicious anemia, 22t, 73, 166f, 202
Phenobarbital (Donnatal), 30t
PillCam. See Capsule endoscopy
   ("PillCam")
Pimecrolimus (Elidel), 160, 202
Platelet (PLT) count, 33
Pneumococcal vaccine, 151, 202
Pneumococcus infection, 151
Potato starch/flour, 202

Potential celiac disease. See Latent
   (potential) CD
Prealbumin, 202
Prednisone, 173, 202
Primary biliary cirrhosis, 22t, 41, 166f,
   202
Primary sclerosing cholangitis, 41,
   166f, 202–203
Probactrix, 153
Probiotics, 152, 153–154, 203
Protein, 2, 203
Protopic (tacrolimus), 160
Psoriasis, 158, 166f 203
Psychiatric and neurological disease,
   18–19, 37–38, 66, 166f
Pyx, 130, 203

Quinoa, 203

Raynaud's phenomenon, 166f
Red blood cell(s) (RBC)
   count, 33–34
   loss of red blood cells (bleeding), 34
   shortened red blood cell lifespan,
      36
Refractory (sprue) CD, 21, 117, 137,
   172–173, 203
Relatives, incidence of CD among,
   6–8, 7t
Resources for patients
   gluten-free alcohol products,
      121–122, 121t
   gluten-free diet, 110, 183t, 184–186
   medical information on CD,
      187–188, 188t
   support groups for celiac patients,
      182–184, 183t
   support or information for children
      with CD, 186–187, 187t
   used in writing the book, 193–194

Restaurants that are celiac-friendly, 122–123, 124–125*t*, 126
Rheumatoid arthritis, 22*t*, 73, 166*f*, 203
Rheumatologic disease associated with CD, 166*f*
Rheumatologist, 40, 203
Rice, 52, 203
Rickets, 39, 203
Rochester Celiac Support (NY), 183*t*
Rye, 2, 3, 203

Sago, 52, 203
Scalloping of the mucosa, 90, 203
Scleroderma, 146, 166*f*, 203
Scopolamine (Scop patch), 30*t*
Scurvy, 203
Second-degree relative, 7, 7*t*
Secretin therapy for autism, 58, 203
Sedimentation rate (ESR), 203
Seitan, 203
Selective IgA deficiency, 203
Selective immunoglobulin A (IgA) deficiency, 22, 22*t*, 56–57, 61–62
    blood testing for, 163
    false-negative blood testing for CD and, 163
    manifestations of, 162
    risk of developing allergic diseases and, 163
    risk of developing autoimmune disease and, 163
    role of in the body, 162
Semolina, 203
Sensitivity of blood tests, 75–76, 75*t*, 203
Sensitivity to gluten, and allergy, compared, 46–47
Sexual impairment, 37
Sicca syndrome, 22*t*, 203

Silent CD
    in children, 53, 54*f*
    definition of, 20, 203
Sjogren's syndrome, 166*f*, 203
    in children, 57
Skin diseases associated with CD, 158*t*, 166*f*
    alopecia areata, 158–159
    dermatitis herpetiformis (DH), 156–160
    eczema, 158
    psoriasis, 158
    vitiligo, 158
Small bowel follow-through, 98–100, 99*f*, 203
Small intestinal lymphoma, 174, 175
    diagnosis of, 99
Small intestine, definition of, 204
Small intestine bacterial overgrowth (SIBO), 44–45, 203
Small intestine biopsy. *See under* Biopsy
Smooth muscle, 29, 204
Sorghum, 204
Soy, 11, 204
Soy milk, 32
Specificity of blood tests, 75–76, 75*t*, 204
Spelt, 204
Spleen
    anemia and, 36
    definition of, 151, 204
Sprue. See Celiac disease (CD)
Starches, gluten-free, 114–115, 114*t*
Steroids, 173, 204
Stools
    appearance of, in persons with CD, 14
    incontinence of, 14
    studies, 100–101

Stores providing gluten-free foods, 119, 120*t*
Stricture, 204
Sulfapyridine (Dapsone), 160, 197
Supplements
    calcium, 40
    enzyme, 32, 111
    gluten-free multivitamins, 114
    iron, 150*t*
    magnesium, 150*t*
    omega-3 fatty acid, 153–154
    thiamine, 150*t*
    vitamin A (carotene), 150*t*
    vitamin and mineral supplements, 63–64
    vitamin B$_{12}$, 150*t*
    vitamin D, 40
    zinc, 150*t*
Support groups for celiac patients, 182–184, 183*t*
Surreptitious consumption of gluten, 20, 115–116, 204
Swedish blood donors, rate of CD among, 6*t*
Symptomatic CD, in children, 54, 54*f*
Symptoms and manifestations of celiac disease
    in adults, 2
    anemia associated with CD, 33–36
        causes of
            abnormal production of red blood cells, 34–36
            loss of red blood cells (bleeding), 34
            shortened red blood cell lifespan, 36
        complete blood count (CBC), 33–34
        general symptoms of, 33
    asymptomatic disease, 21

asymptomatic symptoms
    anemia, 16–17
    arthritis and bone pain, 19
    dermatitis herptiformis (DH), 18
    eczema and other rashes, 18
    generalized, nonspecific symptoms, 18
malnutrition, 19
    muscle abnormalities, 19
    oral manifestations, 18
    osteoporosis, 17–18
    psychiatric and neurological problems, 18–19, 66, 166*f*
bone disease/osteoporosis and CD, 38–40
    evaluation for bone health, 39–40
    low blood calcium levels, 39
    poor absorption of vitamin D, 39
    risk factors, 38–39
    treatments, 39–40
can one have a sensitivity to gluten but not have CD?
    difficulty in diagnosing CD and, 47
    sensitivity and allergy compared, 46–47
cancer and CD, 42–43
in children, 2–3, 15
diarrheal diseases occurring with CD, 43–46
    causes of
        autoimmune thyroid disease, 45
        bile salt diarrhea, 45
        irritable bowel syndrome, 44
        lactose intolerance, 44
        microscopic colitis, 45–46
        small intestine bacterial overgrowth (SIBO), 44–45
    evaluation by a colonoscopy, 45–46

diseases associated with, 21–23, 22*t*

diseases that mimic CD
  bile salt diarrhea, 50
  Crohn's disease, 48
  giardia, 49
  gluten sensitivity, 47
  HIV, 49
  hyperthyroidism, 49
  IBS, 47
  microscopic colitis, 48
  tropical sprue, 48
  tuberculosis, 49
  Whipple's disease, 48

fertility and CD, 36–37

gastrointestinal symptoms, 14–15, 15*t*

irritable bowel syndrome (IBS), 27–30, 30*t*

laboratory and blood abnormalities associated with, 23–24, 24*t*

lactose intolerance
  association with CD, 31
  in certain ethnic groups, 31
  in children, 30–31
  description of, 30
  diagnosis of by a lactose breath test, 31–32
  diagnosis of by its symptoms, 31
  dietetary restrictions, 31
  should all people with it be checked for CD?, 32–33
  treatment, 32

liver abnormalities and CD, 40–42
  testing for, 41–42
  types and causes of liver disease, 40–41

missed diagnoses, 16

most common symptoms, 14

overweight and obese persons and CD, 24–27, 26*f*

severity of disease and, 14

systemic manifestations, 15*t*, 16–19

types of CD based on symptoms, 19–21

T-score, 148, 204

Tacrolimus (Protopic), 160, 204

Tapioca, 204

Teff, 204

Testing. *See* Evaluation and diagnosis

Tetany, 39, 204

Thiamine
  deficiency, 38
  definition of, 204
  role of, 149*t*
  supplementation, 150*t*

Thyroid, definition of, 45, 204

Thyroid disease associated with CD, 22*t*, 45, 49, 166–167

Thyroid test (TSH), 104*t*

Tight junctions, 111, 204

Tissue transglutaminase (tTG) test, 61, 62, 70, 74, 75, 77, 77*t*, 204

Total parenteral nutrition (TPN), 172, 204

Transferrin, 204

Trisomy 21. See Down syndrome

Triticale, 204

Tropical sprue, 9, 48, 204. *See also* Celiac disease (CD)

Tuberculosis, 49, 204

Turner syndrome, 22*t*, 56, 60*t*, 204

Type 1 (juvenile) diabetes
  associated with CD, 22*t*
    in children, 57, 60*t*, 65–66
    delay in diagnosis of CD and risk of diabetes, 163–164
    effects of gluten-free diet, 164
    percentage with CD, 163

screening of diabetics with GI
symptoms, 164
definition of, 204

Ulcerative jejunitis, 173–174
definition of, 205
diagnosis of, 99
symptoms, 141
Undiagnosed CD, 20, 205
University of Chicago Celiac Disease
Program, guidelines for taking
low-gluten host, 130–131
Upper GI series, 98–100, 99f, 205

Vaccinations, 151–152
Vendors of gluten-free foods, 119,
120t
Viactiv, 40
Villi, 2, 3f
definition of, 3, 205
endoscopy samples from, 86
functions of, 91–93, 92f
Vitamin A (carotene)
definition of vitamin A, 205
role of, 149t
supplementation, 150t
testing for, 104, 149t
Vitamin B$_{12}$
ataxia and peripheral neuropathy
and, 38
definition of, 205
malabsorption of by the gut, anemia
and, 34–35
role of, 149t

sources of B$_{12}$ in the diet, 34
supplementation, 150t
tests for, 102, 104t
Vitamin C, 205
Vitamin D
absorption, 21, 39
blood levels, 40, 102–103, 104t
deficiency in children, 64–65, 66t
definition of, 205
role of, 149t
supplementation, 40, 150t
Vitamin K, 145, 205
Vitiligo, 22t, 158, 166f, 205
VSL#3, 152–153, 205

Warfarin (Coumadin), 205
Weight loss in CD, 14–15. *See also*
Obesity and weight gain
with the gluten-free diet, 117
Wheat bran/germ/starch, 205
Wheaton Gluten-Free support group,
107
Whipple's disease, 48, 205
White blood cell (WBC) count, 33
Wichita Celiac Support Group, 183t
Williams syndrome, 22t, 56, 60t, 205

Zinc
deficiency, symptoms of, 65
definition of, 205
role of, 149t
supplementation, 150t
Zometa, 40
Zonulin, 112, 192, 205